The GENETIC KEY Diet

The Key to Unlock a Lean Body & a Long Healthy Life

by Dr. Steve Nugent

Published by *The Alethia Corporation*

To order additional copies of this book, please contact:
Dupli-Pack at 1-888-443-1979 or visit: **www.glycotools.com**

The information in this book is not intended or recommended as a means of diagnosing or treating any physical or mental condition. All matters concerning physical and mental health should be supervised by a health practitioner knowledgeable in treating that particular condition.

Contents

Why should you read this book?

The truth about diets even most doctors don't know
- Low calorie
- Low fat
- Low cholesterol
- Low carbohydrate
- Single food fad diets
- Low Glycemic
- Glycemic Load
- Graphic, statistical and historical evidence that proves the G factor is the only way to lasting success and the healthiest life.

- Why the **Genetic Key Diet** is the best diet for fat loss, prevention of diabetes and prevention of heart disease.

What's your metabolic type?
- The facts about all metabolic-typing systems
- How to find out what metabolic type you are?
- What's the perfect diet for your metabolic type?
- Simple guides for success

What's the reason for increased appetite and how do you control it?
- Three causes, three solutions
- How do nutritional supplements help you to control appetite?
- Nutritional recommendations

Why do you hit plateaus and how to overcome them?
- The thrifty gene
- The metabolic weight set point
- The crucial role of antioxidants

How do I use the Genetic Key Diet ?
- The **Genetic Key Diet** explained
- How to choose the right foods for your type
- Hundreds of foods listed with simple color key
- Daily menus for your **Genetic Key** to success

The truth about exercise and diet, it's not what you think
- No need for a gym, no excuses
- My personal travel fitness program
- The most frequently asked questions answered throughout

Introduction
The last diet you'll ever need

In this book you will learn about the last diet you will need for the rest of your life. If you understand and **follow** the simple guidelines that I have created for you, you will succeed in getting excess body fat off and keeping it off. What you will learn is based on the latest science, but given to you in simple easy everyday language.

I have learned from both my personal experience, as well as in my clinical practice with weight loss patients. Theories are always interesting; but if you can say you've been there and done that, you really have something practical and valuable to offer. Nothing speaks louder than personal experience.

Yes, throughout this book I will give you science (in plain language) and tell you about all the theories (fact and fiction) and, of course, tell you about my clinical experiences with various methods and metabolic types. I want you to have confidence that this diet works; I know because I have been fat and now I'm lean.

My weight loss story
As a young man I was a United States Marine. Talk about exercise! The Marines put the "F" in fitness. The U.S. Marines have something called a PFT or physical fitness test. It's the toughest of all the services with a maximum possible score of 300, I came in at 298. As we used to say; I was a lean, mean, fighting machine. I weighed 215 lbs (97.5 kilograms or 15.4 stone as they say in the UK) and was 6'1" (185.42 centimeters) and I had a 34-inch (86.36 centimeter) waist. I was definitely lean and muscular. It was the best shape I had ever been in. How could I weigh that much and not be fat? Well, I'll explain that later.

In civilian life, between work and graduate school, I became more sedentary. As I got older, my metabolism slowed down. I went on a low fat diet and gained weight. Looking for an answer, I did some research and found that certain foods raise your insulin levels. Hyperinsulin response was first documented in 1979[1] to be associated with obesity in 100% of the cases tested to that time. It's pretty hard to argue with 100% response. That was enough to convince me, all those years ago, that I needed to choose foods that would not raise my insulin levels abnormally. At that time the words low glycemic had not yet been coined.

I was a great admirer of the work of Dr. Roger Williams. His writings made great sense to me, and his work set me a on path to find the **Genetic Key** that would unlock the mechanisms that would lead to safe, effective, and natural fat loss.

So I designed my own diet and didn't have any catchy name for it. It worked in a big way. After I started in clinical practice, it was the diet I recommended most often for my patients, and it worked for them, as well; particularly for certain metabolic types which were identified by serum analysis (blood testing) not blood typing. In all of the patients I put on the diet it brought down high cholesterol, high triglycerides and high blood sugar. It wasn't low fat and it got me continuous grief from referring physicians, who despite the fact that they had failed and my method succeeded with their patients, insisted I was wrong. Why? Well, because "everybody knows" low fat is the correct way to eat, they would say.

I know you've met overweight diet doctors and pulmonary oncologists (lung cancer doctors) who smoke. Well, believe it or not, doctors are human beings. I'm human too. Succumbing to human weakness, I made the same mistake as most people with a slow metabolism; I became sedentary again. My work dominated my life to the point of absolute fatigue each day. I began to answer body's need for energy by eating and drinking quick-fix foods that spiked my insulin, and I began to get fat. As I became fat again, I recommended the diet that I knew worked for everyone, the diet that was the **Genetic Key** to success.

I managed to get myself up to 248 ponds (112.5 kilograms or 17.7 stone) and I was more than 36% body fat. I had a big fluffy 48-inch (121.92 centimeters) waist. It was not a pretty sight, not exactly the picture of health. By using what I now call the **"Genetic Key Diet"**, I unlocked those mechanisms that made me gain and retain weight; I took 10 inches (25.4) off my formerly fluffy waste line using the simple principles you are about to learn. In the process, I reduced my cholesterol, triglycerides (blood fats) and blood pressure as well as normalized my blood sugar. Does that sound desirable to you?

I did this in 1998-1999 and have kept it off to this day. Many thousands of others have had similar success using my method. Some of the success stories since 1999 have been incredible, even tear jerking, as chronically obese people without hope have changed their lives in ways even they could not believe.

The **"Genetic Key Diet"** is not based on short cuts, gimmicks or dangerous substances that interfere with the body's normal processes. This is the most natural thing you can imagine and that is why, <u>if you follow this method as directed</u>, you will succeed for life.

The **"Genetic Key Diet"** is easy once you understand the principles so I will spend a significant part of the book explaining how to do that and shattering all the myths many doctors and laymen still believe to be facts about diet and metabolism. Once I have shown you why people fail on other methods, you can clear your mind of all that nonsense and reset your mental hard drive to think and to eat the way you were designed to. In other words, using your personal **Genetic Key** you can unlock the mechanisms in you that have kept you overweight and out of shape.

If you choose to follow this method and do so faithfully, this truly is the last diet you will ever need to learn about. It's simple, it's safe, it results in true fat loss not just weight loss (I'll explain the difference later) and it works! The latest science also proves it is the best diet not only for fat loss, but it is also the best diet for the prevention of heart disease and diabetes as well.

You will make the choice to be lean, firm and healthy by following the **"Genetic Key Diet"** and having unprecedented success and health, or to reduce your quality of life as well as your life span by continuing to follow other outdated diet methods.

Life is full of choices. I hope you choose wisely.

We need to clear out that outdated intercranial cargo

In 1998 I created the world's first complete system, with dietary supplement support and exercise recommendations specifically designed to work with glycemic index dieting. We launched that system in 1999. Even my friends and colleagues at the time told me I was wrong because "Everybody knows" that low calorie or low fat is the right way to diet. I will prove to you, just as I did to them, that Low cal and Low fat are wrong for almost everyone who has trouble losing weight. Every person is unique with their own personal **Genetic Key** that needs to be accessed and used to achieve true, safe, healthy fat loss. People are not identical products produced on an assembly line that all fit in the same categories with the same treatments and recommendations. No, my friends, we are each wonderfully unique and special. You will soon find that the **"Genetic Key Diet"** is the key to good health and a lean firm, healthy, beautiful body. You were designed to be lean and healthy. It's just a matter of finding your key.

The **"Genetic Key Diet"** involves the glycemic response for each genetic metabolic type with some variations, based on my clinical experience. I will explain in detail what this means later. Our goal is to find and use the **Genetic Key** factor to get you into the **GK** Zone. This is the biochemical zone in which your body metabolizes fat as energy with no harmful and with many healthful effects on your body, based on your genetic factors. It sounds more complex than it is. Relax, you'll find this is incredibly simple.

Why did I choose to call it the **"Genetic Key Diet"**? This diet is based on two primary factors, first biochemical individuality. Second the scientific evidence that proves hyperinsulin responses not fat intake are the primary cause of fat gain and fat retention.[1]

After many years of attempting to teach, under the heading of glycemic indexing and metabolic typing, it has become clear that the words glycemic indexing turn people off. Maybe it sounds too complex. Maybe it simply isn't catchy enough for today's media driven culture. I am not sure, but I know the **Genetic Key** is easy to remember and not intimidating. With all the publicity on genetics over the last ten years, the general public recognizes that genes play a key role in who we are and how healthy we are. Whereas the majority of the public still doesn't know what glycemic indexing is.

Additionally, others have written about the glycemic index since Dr. Jenkins invented it, but each author seems to have their own variation of the theme. I have learned from many years of experience that calculating the glycemic index or even the glycemic load is not enough for some to succeed. So the **"Genetic Key Diet"** has additional components over and above those two important concepts to find your key to long-term success and true optimal health.

Before I introduced my dietary system for glycemic index dieting in 1999, I had already learned much in my many years of clinical experience about the psychology of diet and why people fail on diets. However, after launching that system I learned much more about the questions and misconceptions the general public has regarding dieting.

To my dismay, I found that many people did not read any of the material I wrote to support the system. Many assumed it was simply what they incorrectly thought low carb was. They mixed and matched principles with systems they had failed on before or heard about and, of course, never found their Genetic Keys. So this book will put all the pieces together for you. For this reason I strongly recommend you read the entire book. I know that's a lot to ask of some people, but please be patient and do this. I have made this book short, to the point, and simple to read. I have deliberately written this not as a science or textbook, but as something anyone can understand and succeed with. If you are going to succeed you must concentrate only on using the principles of the **"Genetic Key Diet"** to get you into the GK Zone.

Gimmicks always fail
Books that sell well are those that take incredibly complex issues and simplify them to one thought, one phrase, or one cause. That's how authors in the alternative or complementary health care area become rich and famous. They take complex disease mechanisms, for which there is no proven answer, and blame all of them on a single thing that laymen can relate to and blissfully embrace as a fact. Such as, all health problems known are due to candida or parasites etc. That is nice, convenient, easy and... almost always incorrect.

Many authors have done the same for diets. Diet books simply don't sell well unless they have a catchy name and a single food type, food category or gimmick. There have been zillions of them come and go and there will be zillions more, despite my efforts. Those who have tried those flash in the pan systems "may" have had short-term success but long-term failure. After using the gimmick diets, typically they end up with worse health problems and more difficulty with weight management.

So I won't say just eat one kind of food for "X" number of days. That is unnatural; it goes against your genetic design, and that is why those gimmick diets always fail long-term. I hope the name of the diet is easy to remember but there are a significant number of factors and principles to making it work. The minimalist approach is often counterproductive and even potentially harmful. My approach is to explain all the facts objectively and completely, and then, once you understand those facts, give you quick simple summaries to your personal **Genetic Key,** to speed you on the road to success.

The **"Genetic Key Diet"** works with your body, not against it and you'll be surprised how good health follows this system. My life's goal is to help as many people worldwide with their health as I can everyday. A key component to being truly healthy is being lean, that is to say low levels of body fat. So, understand that The **"Genetic Key Diet"** is about fat loss yes, but it is the right way for all human beings to eat for the prevention of heart disease and diabetes as well. With this in mind it is far more than a fat loss system. [1,2,3,4,5,6,7,8,9,10,11,12,13]

My writing style
You'll find that my writing style is somewhat unique. That's because I am first a public speaker. For more than thirty years, I have spoken to live audiences numbering into the hundreds of thousands, and radio and TV audiences numbering into the millions in many countries. Those who have heard my lectures and classes around the world can hear my voice as they read my books, and I like it that way. I want you to feel that I am with you in spirit, helping you on

every step of this new and important journey to optimal health.

A Real Book
It has been my experience that few people these days will take the time to completely read a lengthy, detailed book. I could easily write several hundred pages on the subject of diet, metabolism and healthy eating in general. In fact, it is very difficult for me to condense this information in a piece this short. So I had to make a decision. Do I write about everything I want you to know and have a several hundred page, highly-detailed book that only a very small percentage of people will read; or do I want to write a brief concise, easy-to-read piece that can put you on the right path for your health quickly and that the vast majority of people will read? As you can see by what you are holding in your hands, I chose the later. This book may be criticized for not being the "War and Peace" of diet books. Call this text what you will, but know that it delivers the vital information you need in a simple, easy, and brief format. There is no excuse for not reading this text in its entirety.

Deliberate redundancy
I will be deliberately redundant in some areas because despite what I have just said, experts tell us that many people will misquote or misunderstand what they have read even though they saw it in print. Coupled with the fact that some of these concepts are so different from what most people have learned before, that some readers may need to have the thoughts reinforced several times before they really understand.

Psychologists tell us that the average person has to hear or see something between 7 and 27 times before they fully understand and can utilize the information. Second, some people will not read the entire text, but rather look for that information that they believe to be most necessary to them. With this in mind, there are sections of this book that almost stand alone as their own booklets.

Absolutes
You will also find that unlike other authors, I work hard to avoid absolutism and subjective thought. The always or never psychology (absolutism) and using subjective thinking to arrive at conclusions has caused more misery to humanity than any single thing in history in my opinion. Pre-judging or using subjective thinking is often called prejudice. Jumping to conclusions before you have examined "all" sides of an issue, even those you are uncomfortable with, is nearly always not only wrong, it most often leads to a negative net result.

It is unfortunately human nature (though there are a few exceptions) to want to think and speak in absolutes. It makes life easier and reduces psychological stress by doing so, because we don't have to think about the complex mind-bending issues that confront us everyday.

In today's world psychological stress has reached new heights and information overload has made most of us want to seek the quick, simple, and easy. When it comes to the complex workings of the human body however there are very few things which we can put under the headings of always or never. Diet is no different.

So please try not to draw conclusions before you are done reading the complete text.

Having said all that, rest assured that the ideas you read in this book will be expressed in the simplest and easiest possible terms with frequent simple summaries.

The GENETIC KEY Diet

SECTION 1

The History of Diets

The Key to Unlock a Lean Body & a Long Healthy Life

by Dr. Steve Nugent

Chapter 1

This first chapter covers the brief history of diet and the calorie theory with its effects on our population. The next two chapters will cover low fat and low carb dieting.

Some definitions you'll need before reading further

Metabolic weight set point theory: this theory says that all of us have a particular metabolic type based on our genetic makeup. It further states that we each have a set point at which our body wants to store fat to avoid starvation. This is the point at which many plateau on diets.

The Thrifty Gene: first discovered in 1962, the theory in simple terms says, we have a genetic trigger that will slow our rate of fat burn and perhaps stop fat burn (be thrifty and save fat) in order to prevent starvation.[12]

Insulin: a hormone made by the pancreas to normalize high blood sugar.

Hyperinsulin response: when your pancreas is forced to secrete abnormally large levels of insulin to bring down unusually high blood sugar levels. According to studies, this is always associated with obesity. [1]

Glycemic: derived from the Greek word glukus, which means sweet-used now to refer to the effects that any food has on blood sugar.

Glycemic index: a numerical value that shows the effect on blood sugar when you consume a given food.

The GK factor: refers to the glycemic index, the glycemic load and the glucagon mechanism and your personal **Genetic Key** with my personal clinical variations to get you into the **GK Zone**.

Glucagon is a hormone that is produced by the pancreas. It raises blood sugar levels by promoting the conversion of glycogen into glucose in the liver. Gluco refers to blood sugar and agon is the Greek word meaning, to lead.

Glucagon mechanism: the process by which this hormone selects to store what you have eaten as fat or burn it for energy. Hyperinsulin responses cause this mechanism to select fat storage rather than fat burn.

The GK Zone: the zone at which we burn excess fat and maintain normal blood sugar and prevent coronary artery disease and diabetes.

Low G foods: low glycemic foods, will not trigger a hyperinsulin response or any of the negatives associated with it, including weight gain. Foods that are low glycemic and have a low glycemic load are Low G.

Moderate G foods: moderate glycemic foods may trigger a hyperinsulin response or any of the negatives associated with it in some individuals depending on metabolic type.

High G foods: High glycemic foods will trigger a hyperinsulin response and contribute to the negatives associated with it, but only triggers weight gain in some metabolic types.

The History Of Diets, A History Of Failure
"Those who cannot learn from history are doomed to repeat it."
George Santayana, Philosopher, poet 1863-1886
So let's learn the history so we don't have to repeat it with our diets.

Here is the Chronology
- First recorded low carb diet 1860
- First diet movement 1898 (reduced food consumption and increased cereals)
- Calorie theory USA 1930
- Low Carbohydrate USA 1960's
- Dr. Atkins Diet Revolution 1972
- American Diet Craze Starts 1972
- Hyperinsulinism and obesity connection, Canada 1979
- Glycemic Index invented, Canada 1981[2]
- Low Fat, USA 1980s*
- Low Glycemic, Australia and Canada 1990's
- Low Glycemic, USA 1997 (Harvard Medical School only)
- Low Glycemic makes front page USA Today March 2005

Why do we need a dramatic paradigm shift from old failed methods? Because:
In America there are 295,734,134 million people as of July 2005
- **105 million have cholesterol above 200 mg/dl (high)**
- **73 million have high blood pressure**
- **61 million are obese**
- **17 million have diabetes**
- **More than 90 million do not exercise at all**

Considering that Americans spend more money on weight loss than any people in the world per capita, America is without a doubt the most dismal failure, in terms of weight loss, of any country in the world. Every country who adopts America's foods and diet methods becomes fatter and unhealthier every year. Do you think there is a clue there? Even Japan is having the first significant increase in history with weight gain and diabetes. The World Health Organization is already calling diabetes the fastest growing disease on planet Earth. In fact experts believe that at the current rate, adult onset of Type 2 diabetes will double worldwide by the year 2025.[14,15,16,17] If we don't learn from our mistakes and begin to teach people to eat in truly healthy ways, the numbers in these categories will simply get worse every year in every country.

Now I would like to call your attention to the first map in the center of the book. This shows the rankings from the World Health Organization of which countries have the greatest percentage of people who are overweight. Hmm... Look who's number one, the country that invented Low Cal, Low Fat and Low Carbohydrate dieting.

There are, of course, many factors that contribute to this alarming fact, but the point is that the US is the most miserable failure in terms of weight management in the world. That has to say something about the recommended methods of dieting by US so-called experts. We can also see from this history that science moves very slowly from the time an idea or theory is conceived, to the time it is finally accepted as fact.

In the center of the book you will find some maps that show statistics kept by the United States Centers for Disease Control (CDC). I will refer to these maps again later but for now let me explain what they show.

Starting in 1962 the CDC began keeping records of the percentage of US citizens who were overweight and obese. Up until 1980 there was no statistically significant change in the level of obesity in the total of the US population while low cal was the popular method of dieting. However in the 80's after low fat was introduced, there was a jump in the level of obesity in the US by almost 10%. [16]

Why didn't anyone notice this trend? Why did all the authorities ignore the massive data that showed low fat foods, (which were also high glycemic) were causing weight gain, and the other methods had no major effect on the population at all? I'll give more detail when we discuss cholesterol mania and the low fat fad. First, let's talk about the various diet methods in the order they were introduced and why they fail for most dieters.

The History of Caloric dieting
US scientists at the University of Michigan invented low calorie dieting in 1930. So, Low cal dieting isn't exactly new or cutting edge. Yet, it was universally adapted by medical schools around the planet by 1931, and believed to be simple and fool-proof for all. Guess what? It isn't.

Do Calories count?
Of course they do, but not in the way you think. Although in a strict sense a calorie is a calorie, it must be understood that calories do not reflect nutritional value but rather a unit of energy. The nutritional value from 1000 calories provided by vegetables (low G foods) and the nutritional value provided by 1000 calories from candy (high G foods) are going to be vastly different. Just reducing calories alone will not necessarily reduce your fat or contribute to a healthier body, unless the calories chosen are from the right foods. This is one of the reasons that many have failed on low calorie diets.

Candy is high glycemic; the insulin stress on the body is obvious. Most vegetables are low glycemic so they not only provide superior nutrition per calorie they also provide health-supporting fiber and do not contribute to blood sugar imbalances, diabetes or heart disease. Low glycemic foods also increase long-term stamina and help to reduce appetite. There have been patients who on reduced calorie diets had little or no success in fat loss because they were not choosing the right calories to restrict. Other factors such as the weight set point and metabolic type also played a role.

1000 calories from broccoli is low glycemic = no hyperinsulin response
1000 calories from white bread is high glycemic = hyperinsulin response

Clearly starvation will eventually reduce anyone's weight, but reducing calories without considering the glycemic index will cause the body to burn muscle as food before it burns fat as food. This is because there is far more nutrition in muscle than in fat. I'll come back to that concept later.

Yes, if you eat more calories than you need you will store the excess and if you eat fewer calories than you need you should theoretically, or at least eventually, loose stored body fat; but it isn't that simple for two of the five metabolic types. Moreover, you have a survival mechanism in your brain, called the weight set point that monitors not just caloric intake but also nutrient intake; and if it senses a food shortage, it will reduce the rate at which you convert stored fat into energy. It does this because the Thrifty Gene is triggered and it makes you save fat to save your life. So, your metabolism slows down and at some point you will plateau. Your body's first priority is survival, not fitting into your favorite swim suit.

So yes, if you starve yourself enough, you will eventually loose weight; but after you return to your old habits again, you will gain back on average (according to statistics) at least 25% more weight than you lost. To make this scenario a little bit worse, the next time you diet it will be harder than the last time. Your body doesn't want to let you starve. Even though high G calories cause a hyperinsulin response and therefore a dysfunction of the glucagon mechanism, at a certain level of starvation there will be no more fat to save.

Last, there is the issue of metabolic types. Later I'll explain what they are, how they affect you, and how you determine yours. Some types can eat enormous calories and not gain weight. But if those calories are from high glycemic foods, they will still stress their pancreas and hasten their journey towards adult onset diabetes, as well as, produce triglycerides to clog their arteries and promote heart disease. Think about it, you know thin diabetics and thin people who have had heart attacks, don't you? High glycemic food is bad for everyone, whether it causes you to increase body fat or not.

Chapter 2
Low Carbohydrate is definitely not new

To be accurate, we would have to say that low carb was invented in the 60's... the 1860's. An Englishman, William Banting, decided to take action (as the story goes) when he became too fat to bend over and tie his own shoes. A letter exists called "Letter on Corpulence," written by Banting that advocated avoiding starch and sugar. He lost 45 pounds on a diet of lean meat, dry toast, soft boiled eggs, and a few alcoholic drinks a day. Yes, most alcohol is Low G. Nobody else seemed to like his diet despite his obvious success. What happened to him later? Did he gain it back? We don't know. Was the famous Dr. Atkins influenced by old Bill Banting? I guess we'll never know the answer to that question either.

Those of us old enough to remember may recall that there were people low carb dieting in the late sixties. Yes, that's right, and the younger you are the more likely you are to think that it's new. Dr. Atkins was doing Low carb with his patients starting in 1960, but it was in 1972 that Dr. Atkins took the country (and eventually the world) by storm with his first of many books on High Protein Low Carbohydrate dieting. Although many attempts had been started at diet trends, he really was the catalyst for the American diet craze. People would try what they thought was his diet, lose fast, get bored with the menu, go back to their old high glycemic habits and gain the weight back plus additional fat weight because the imbalance triggered their Thrifty Genes.[12] A few years later, an update to one or more of his books would be introduced and a new generation would think it was a totally new diet concept. I have met some young people who think it's a new diet as of 2005.

Dr. Atkins once told me that one of his biggest frustrations was that almost no one who claimed to be on his diet had actually read any of his books to fully understand his intent. Before the initial research on glycemic indexing was done in 1981, Dr. Atkins was unknowingly, to some degree, leaning in that direction; but it didn't quite hit the mark. Before his untimely death, he was beginning to work the glycemic index into his system. Eventually, he would have gained support from much of the scientific community as a result of doing that, but like many famous men he didn't live long enough to enjoy that.

The real excitement about the diet for the general public was that it seemed so easy and the results were, for many, incredibly fast. The problem is if you simply restrict carbohydrates without regard for the glycemic index and balanced nutrition, you will cause your body to trigger its innate protection mechanisms.

I do not believe it was ever Dr. Atkins intent for people to eat red meat all day everyday for the rest of their lives, yet the masses thought it was and off they went on a very unhealthy path.

A 100% protein and fat diet is not the natural way for your body to function; and because people did not follow that diet correctly, many had health issues. By eating this highly imbalanced way, you trigger the thrifty gene as well as the body's genetic nutrition mechanisms. Balance is the key to wellness. So although many enjoyed very rapid and tremendous success on this diet, it eventually back-fired on them. I watched many patients, including one of my closest loved ones who wouldn't listen to me, have huge exciting rapid success only to have it all reverse later. Eventually she found that she had to keep reducing the carbs daily to maintain weight and eventually at 0 grams of carbohydrates per day was gaining fat! I saw one individual who had lost 120 pounds in 14 months then gain back 145 pounds in 8 months. Without balance, you will pay a price; short-term success is simply not worth the long-term penalty.

Further confusion regarding the low carb diet resulted in endless criticism of Dr. Atkins by the mainstream medical community. Medical doctors had been taught before Atkins that low fat was the right way to diet. Some doctors were on to that theory or a version of it as early as 1948 when the famous Framingham study, which continues today, was first started.

Once again, absolutes misdirected everyone from doctors to laymen. Many researchers were saying and teaching that fat makes fat and mislead the public into thinking that cholesterol was fat or vice versa. They assumed if you ate fat you got fat and heart disease. Some of the misinformed still do. So they attacked Atkins and low carb dieting because they saw it as an absolute. To them, Atkins was a high fat diet and that meant heart disease. When we cover low fat I'll explain the real facts behind that. For now, I'll just say that if you combine a high fat, food with a high G food you will get heart disease, but because of the high G food <u>not the high fat food</u>.

Carbohydrates, just like calories, have to be selected by their glycemic index in order to get into and stay in the GK Zone. Just as calories from high glycemic foods have an adverse affect on the G factor, so do carbohydrates from high glycemic foods. I will discuss foods and show you a chart of high, moderate, and low G foods, along with an explanation of how to select them and continue your success later.

Before I give you the example, here is a reminder and a word of caution.

Remember what I said about thinking in absolutes and drawing conclusions before you know all the facts? Please keep that in mind. Read the section on food selection before you jump to any conclusions. This example is simply to help you understand that the G Factor diet is not a low carb diet. Here is a brief example.

One example of why the Genetic Key Diet is not a low carb diet
On the **"Genetic Key Diet"** I want you to eat carbohydrates. This is essential to your health and long-term success. But it is essential you avoid high G carbohydrates. Later you will learn all my simple easy GK Rules for getting you in and keeping you in the GK Zone. There are 7 rules that you will learn about soon, but for this example Rules 2 and 3 apply.

GK Rule 2: Eat foods that are comparatively difficult (not impossible) to digest. Humans are only capable of digesting a maximum of 7 % of vegetable fiber if their digestion is perfect, and almost no one has perfect digestion. So fiber is comparatively difficult to digest, and it slows the rate of conversion of the carbohydrates into blood sugar. That's why fiber is low glycemic and will help you stay in the GK Zone.

GK Rule 3: Choose foods that are higher in fiber. For example, white potatoes have virtually no fiber, and sweet potatoes are high in fiber.

A white potato and a sweet potato both have carbohydrates. But a white potato is high G and will push you out of the GK Zone. A sweet potato is low G, and will help you maintain a balance to your diet by giving you necessary carbohydrates while helping you stay in the GK Zone. If you don't have carb intake, your metabolic weight set point and thrifty gene will kick in and all that you achieved will be lost. When I explain the GK Zone and food selection later it will all make sense; but for now just understand that the **"Genetic Key Diet"** is balanced and includes some pretty tasty carbohydrates. Oh, I know if you are having a weight issue, you love white potatoes. Well, my friends there's one reason you are failing on other diets, or you are overweight now. I'll talk more about white potatoes later.

The **"Genetic Key Diet"** selects only low G carbohydrates for the two metabolic types that have the most difficult time with weight management and moderate G with Low G carbohydrates for the other types. Metabolic types will be explained in that chapter, so don't get impatient.

Chapter 3
Low fat dieting and cholesterol mania

Low fat dieting was introduced as a result of the studies done on heart disease and cholesterol in the early seventies to the general public, but really picked up steam in the early eighties as the media started jumping on the bandwagon. Really we could say that the first thoughts regarding cholesterol and heart disease was an after thought of the first year of the now-famous Framingham study, which is on going and began in 1948. Once again, not the newest technology, and it was never the right technology for weight loss for everyone. The amount of misinformation and misunderstanding on fat grams and weight management as well as fat grams and heart disease, is enormous. Once again, I would refer you to the CDC maps at the center of the book.

The Framingham Heart Study gets its name from the town in Massachusetts where it began with 5,000 test subjects. American scientists were concerned about the alarming rate of heart disease, which by the 1940's, was reaching near epidemic proportions. The scientists running the Framingham study said in 1948, that it was due to high blood pressure, cigarette smoking, and high blood cholesterol-in that order. Over the decades cholesterol became the focus, but I believe the more recent facts gathered in the last ten years tells a different story.[4,5,6,7,8,9,10,13] As long as the pharmaceutical companies make obscene amounts of money from selling cholesterol-lowering drugs, they will continue to promote cholesterol as the single most important risk factor. The facts tell us, however, that it is really about individual genetic and hyperinsulin response; it truly is the **Genetic Key,** not fat grams.

Remember from 1962 until the 1980 survey there was no statistically significant change in the level of obesity in the total of the US population while low cal or low carbohydrate were the popular methods of dieting. However, after low fat became the most popular diet there was a jump in the level of obesity in the US by almost 10%, shown on the next national survey. Were the proponents of low fat so sure of themselves that they didn't see what was actually going on? Then the "Everybody knows" mentality kicked in... until now.

Let's take a look at the maps at the center of the book that show the trends over the years, state by state. Look at the first map of the U.S. It shows some states in white where complete data was not available. The rest of the states did report and the darker the color, the greater the percentage of obesity in that state. In 1988, the U.S. had been using low fat and doctors were being taught to recommend low fat for nearly ten years. Is this suspicious? Could low fat but high G foods be increasing obesity?

Now look at the next map of data reported in 1992. Four more years of reinforcing that low fat was the right way to eat and the number of U.S. citizens who are overweight is dramatically higher. I will explain why in a moment.

Now, look at the map from 2000. The percentage overweight of U.S. citizens has increased by an astounding level. By this point in time, virtually anyone you ask would have said; "Yes, everybody knows that low fat is the right way to eat". In fact, in 2004 I saw Jay Leno (a popular American late night TV show host) interview overweight people at random on the streets. Each obese person that he talked with said the best way to eat was low fat; and, in fact, most of them said they were eating low fat. These unfortunate souls were doing what they thought and "everybody knows" is correct and getting fatter and unhealthier with every bite.

Speaking of 2004, let's look at the map from that year, which is the latest data available at this time. What's going on? The more Americans are thinking and eating low fat, the fatter we get as a nation. It's not about fat...it's about the **Genetic Key**. Let's get at the truth of this.

Why not just count fat grams?
There have been writers who discounted fat grams completely in favor of various diet schemes but this is a mistake. Fat grams do count (as do calories), and no one should be loading saturated fat into their diets. Some fats are required for a healthy body, however, in fact, some fats (essential fatty acids) actually help you to convert stored fat as energy. Fat is required for nerve cells and brain cells, so zero fat diets are bad for your health. The key to good health is always balance. The desire to think in absolutes and follow hugely imbalanced diets nearly always backfires on your long-term health.

Saturated fats do present a serious hazard to your health when consumed in high levels, particularly, in conjunction with high G foods. There have also been many who have failed on restricted fat gram diets because once again this is an imbalance and not the diet intended for human physiology. Every person is genetically and biochemically unique; therefore, results and reactions do vary. A common mistake is to look at isolated results that fit the theory of your choice and then declare that the method is absolutely correct.

The real problem is that's exactly the way scientific study works. When a study is done, it is very rarely comprehensive on more than one thought or one question. So often a published study gives us a micro view from inches away but fails to look at the view from 30,000 feet, as the saying goes. With this in mind, frequently a study is published on one fraction of an issue the media gets a hold of, thinks it's the absolute comprehensive last word (because they don't know how studies are done), and then <u>unintentionally</u> misleads the public.

Low fat diets **<u>do not</u>** work for all metabolic types, and in some cases it actually causes fat gain as well as ill health. How can this be? It is because low fat diets often recommend foods that are high G. Remember high G foods raise blood sugar, and that can cause the liver to produce blood fats (triglycerides) and eventually cholesterol which is about 70% triglyceride.[13]

The body does this as an ancient survival mechanism. If fats are not available, the body converts carbohydrates into fats because the body needs a certain amount of fats to be healthy. Unfortunately, in two metabolic types (GK4 and GK5) you will learn that the survival mechanism works too well, and high G carbohydrates become fats virtually all the time. It works in all 5 types, but to a lesser extent in types GK3, GK1 and GK2. That will all be explained later. Be patient, please.

Don't get confused about triglycerides, there are good or energy triglycerides too. The good ones are called medium chain triglycerides, which are absorbed differently and utilized as energy rather than converted to fat. Those are the fats wanted by athletes for energy. An excess of them may still be a problem, however if you are not active enough to burn them up as energy.

As you will see, fat grams are included in a healthy diet, as are calories and carbohydrates; but differently than you may have seen them before. As we look at the data from those maps, we must also reflect on the food manufacturing trends. Food companies want to make a profit on the latest trends (most companies do). So they began by making a mind-boggling variety of low fat foods. The foods that you can buy pre-packaged tend to be primarily high G foods. They tend to be the highest profit foods that have the most marginal nutritional values. The human body was not designed to eat refined pre-packaged foods, no matter how much we enjoy them. We are designed to eat fresh, raw, natural foods, not the high G trash modern society has come to love.

So, many people on low fat diets are eating low fat but high G foods, and the net result is an increase in fat, hanging on the body and/or in the arteries and an increase in diabetes that follow the trend of the consumption of these high G foods. In fact, as of the time of this printing, the World Health Organization says the fastest growing disease on planet Earth is diabetes. I believe the data shows us that this is due to the human population changing their diets to high G foods. At this point some readers are confused, no doubt. So let's look at two examples before we move on.

A white potato is high G, but low fat.
Most breads and cereals (not all) are high G, but low fat.

I'll show some that are not high G later.

Nearly every prepackaged convenience food that is carbohydrate based is made of high G carbohydrates rather than low or moderate G carbohydrates, particularly those advertised as low fat.

Yes, you will learn fat is 0 glycemic, but fat grams must be incorporated into the diet. There must be balance! I say this because I know that there will be some people who will either not read this entire book, or who will not, for whatever reason, understand what they read. When you get to the menu section of the book, you'll see this diet is balanced and includes fat grams and carbohydrate grams. This is not as simple as saying you should eat only red meat all day or only lettuce all day, but it really isn't tough to understand or follow, as you'll soon learn.

The Genetic Key Diet

The GENETIC KEY Diet

SECTION 2

Pounds or Inches?

The Key to Unlock a Lean Body & a Long Healthy Life

by Dr. Steve Nugent

Chapter 4
Is your weight really relevant?

The number of pounds that you weigh is one of the markers for healthy body composition. But it is a marker that has been misunderstood and highly over-rated. Individuals that are very muscular typically weigh more than the medical charts allow for them to weigh for their height and still be healthy. But, of course, their weight is more muscle than fat, and the medical and insurance charts assume that the weight is always more fat mass than muscle mass. Insurance companies always assume the worst-case scenario, which is why they don't lose money.

Muscle tissue is dense and heavy. In fact, muscle weighs approximately three times as much per inch than fat does. Fat tissue is comparatively light and fluffy. Fat tissue takes up far more inches by weight than does muscle. So, the first and most important factor in healthy body composition is the percentage of body fat and, secondly, the number of inches you are above the norm for your height and bone structure. Least in importance is the number of pounds that you weigh. That's worth repeating, the least important factor is how many pounds you weigh so get that thought out of your mind right now.

With healthy body composition, you may in fact weigh more than the medical charts would say is a healthy weight for you; but, if your percentage of body fat is at a healthy level, then you will be healthier and more energetic. The greater your muscle mass, the more easily and efficiently your body burns fat as food so the more you can eat without gaining new inches of fatty deposits. Yes, that's one of the reasons body builders eat more and gain less.

There is also the issue of water weight. Most people don't realize how heavy water actually is. If, as an example, you were to drink the standard/typical rec-ommendation of eight 8-ounce glasses of water each day, you could displace a significant amount of inches. In fact, just in terms of translating the mathemati-cal equation, 64 ounces of fluid can displace as many as 115 cubic inches of vol-ume. Don't panic because each type of tissue in the body absorbs and utilizes water in different amounts and in different ways. So, you won't become a 115 cubic inches larger. You, of course, pass the fluid through you and retain only what you need for hydration. I gave you this example simply to show that water can cause you, not only to gain weight, but also inches. It is temporary and vital-ly important weight, however, because water is the elixir of life.

There is also the matter of scale weight. A U.S. gallon of water weighs 8.4 pounds or 3.818 kilos. If you have consumed the eight 8-ounce glasses of fluid per day, as is typically recommended, you would have gained 4.2 pounds. But the 4.2 pounds are not fat pounds -- this is temporary weight. For this reason, it is a big mistake to get on the scale every day. Your weight will vary literally throughout the day. You will always weigh more at night and less in the morning.

Your weight will vary after each meal. Your weight will increase if you sit down and have a cup of tea, or your 8-ounce glass of water. Your weight varies during your sleep as well. All human beings burn some amount of fat while they sleep, by the way, but for most of us, it simply isn't enough.
Typically, because you lose fluid through perspiration throughout each day, and especially while you sleep, you will weigh less in the morning than you do in the evening.

Scale weight is a very poor, inaccurate, and inefficient way to measure your progress on any diet system. And it's a sure fire way to discourage yourself and give yourself a reason to stop eating right. That's when the person who really doesn't want to succeed says, "Well since I gained weight, I may as well go back to eating unhealthy, until the next diet idea comes around." You can always find excuses to fail; don't let your scale weight be one of them.

The Body Mass Index
Let's discuss BMI or Body Mass Index. The BMI is becoming a popular way internationally for measuring healthy body composition. We need a way to track our progress and this is something that anyone can do without seeing a doctor or being immersed in a chamber to test for body fat. First, I'll explain how it works and then I'll tell you why it doesn't work for everyone.

This is how you calculate your BMI in both U.S. .and metric.

> **U.S.:**
> Multiply your weight (in pounds) by 704.5.
> Multiply your height (in inches) by your height (in inches).
> Divide the first result by the second.
>
> Example: If you're 5'5" and weigh 140:
> 140 x 704.5 = 98,630
> 65 x 65 = 4,225
> 98, 630 divided by 4,225 = 23

Metric:
Multiply your weight (in kilograms) by 10,000.
Multiply your height (in centimeters) by your height (in centimeters).
Divide the first result by the second.

Example: If you're 165 centimeters and weigh 63.6 kilograms:

63.6 x 10,000 =636,000
165 x 165 = 27,225
636, 000 divided by 27,225 = 23.4

This formulation was developed under the same belief as the medical weight charts and that is, that the majority of excess body weight will be fat unless, of course, you adopt a low G lifestyle. Remember the example of a person who is more muscular than average? That person will weigh more then the medical charts allow and some body builders would then be classified by those charts as obese but, of course, they would not be fat.

There is a similar problem with the BMI. It assumes that the amount over the norm is mostly fat, but this is not always the case, particularly with the small but growing number of people who are beginning to work out on a regular basis. In my own case, for example, since I started putting myself into the GK Zone and working out,   I went from 36% body fat to 16.4% body fat in 11 months. I lost a significant amount of pounds but as my body fat continued to decrease and my muscle mass continued to increase, I actually gained healthy pounds. I lost many inches on my waist and elsewhere while doing this. Now if I use the BMI calculation it is nearly 10 points higher than my actual percent of body fat. Had I used the BMI calculation before beginning my fitness program it would have been fairly accurate.

Having said all that, I would suggest you return to the original recommendation of percent body fat and inches.

When you start on the system, weigh yourself the first day. Then, using a tailor's tape, measure the appropriate areas of the body. Once a week, re-measure each area. Measure your progress in inches, not pounds. If you wish to weigh yourself, do so no more frequently than once per week and only first thing in the morning. Even then, scale weight is still not a very accurate gauge of healthy body composition.

Weight loss plans that advertise weight loss as much as a pound a day, or ten pounds a week, are plans that are clearly not measuring fat loss. It will be almost physiologically impossible to lose more than two pounds of <u>pure body fat</u> per seven-day period. There may be rare exceptions but they will be rare indeed. If you are losing more than that, then you are displacing water, and perhaps cannibalizing muscle tissue as fuel. And in some cases, you may also lose bone mass on diets, if these diets are not properly balanced and have the proper dietary supplements. Bone is highly nutritious, not as nutritious as muscle but more nutritious than fat so the body will eat muscle, bone, then fat, in that order when it's starving for nutrients.

One of the most notable cases is a woman who had tremendous success using my system and has lost more than 250 pounds! She lost an average of 1.7 pounds per week. This is excellent. It's healthy, and it's primarily fat. And losing fat is the goal, not losing weight. By the way, that woman had been chronically obese all her life; she unfortunately is a metabolic type GK 5. She had tried every diet and every gimmick known; she had even undergone the now controversial intestinal by-pass surgery. Post the surgery, she did experienced short term dramatic success but gained it all back and much more because she was eating low fat but high G foods. High G foods are bad for everyone's health, but if you are a type GK 4 or GK 5 do not expect to have long-term success if you choose to eat them.

	Inches or centimeters	Week 1	Week 2	Week 3	Week 4	Net Loss
Neck						
Shoulders						
Chest						
Upper arms						
Forearms						
Wrists						
Waist						
Hips						
Thighs						
Calves						
ankles						

The GENETIC KEY Diet

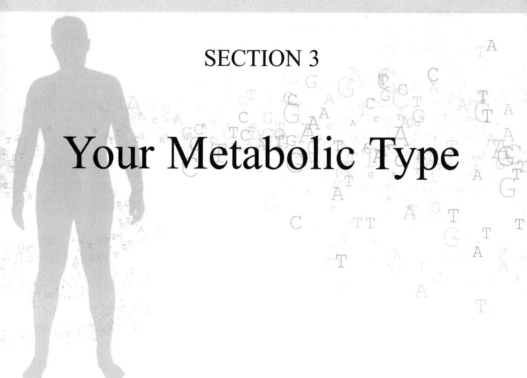

SECTION 3

Your Metabolic Type

The Key to Unlock a Lean Body & a Long Healthy Life

by Dr. Steve Nugent

Chapter 5
What is your metabolic type?

What you will learn in this chapter at a glance

Seven Methods for finding your metabolic type
1. The facts about all Metabolic-typing systems
   a. Serum analysis
   b. Serum Protein electrophoresis
   c. Pheno Types
   d. Blood Type
   e. Body Type
   f. Nervous System Type
2. What is your metabolic type?
3. What's the perfect diet for your metabolic type?
4. Simple guides for success

Finding Your Metabolic Type

Each one of us is genetically and biochemically unique.
Eating right and getting not just nutritional supplementation, but **the right nutritional supplementation**, are essential to achieving and maintaining optimal health.

With individual uniqueness foremost in mind, I developed a simple Genetic Key Survey (GKS) to help you make the best choices about your diet and supplements. This is a variation of a tool I developed for an international dietary supplement company. This self-assessment survey will:

Help you select the diet most appropriate to your individual characteristics so that you can enjoy optimal health.

Help you be aware of and understand many of your individual traits, as well as those you share with other people in your general physical group.

Most important of all, it will serve as your comprehensive guide for making the healthiest lifestyle choices for long-term wellness.

This is designed to increase overall self-knowledge. It will help anyone who uses it become aware of and understand specific nutrition choices we recommend to help them achieve their long-term body composition and wellness goals.

The first step is to determine your body type by completing the survey. Then, after totaling your survey score, you'll read *in easy-to-understand language* about the typical characteristics of your type, the most recommended foods for people in your group, and some information on dietary supplements that should offer you the greatest benefits.

While the GKS is based on the most current health and science research findings, users should understand that this tool is designed to serve as a general set of guidelines and <u>not as a replacement for a properly trained physician's advice</u>.

Evidence of biochemical individuality

In order to understand the metabolic typing concept and to help you understand your metabolic type, it is important for us to first discuss the evidence of biochemical individuality.

Over time, all genetic groups of humans have had to adapt to their environments or face extinction. Only a few genetic groups are left in the world that have maintained their original genetic line, and that is due only to their relative isolation from the rest of humanity. Those groups have given us valuable data about the human body's ability to adapt. That information has broadened our understanding of metabolic types and why certain foods are best for certain people.

I have based much (not all) of my research on hunter-gatherer tribes to ascertain the information you need to find your metabolic type. So, first I'd better define what a hunter-gatherer is. As I have lectured, literally around the world, I have found to my surprise, that many people have no idea what I mean when I say hunter-gatherer. Currently this term is used to describe people who still live in the Stone Age as our ancestors once did. Stone Age makes no reference to time or the theory of evolution necessarily, but rather describes people who use technology no more sophisticated than stone tools. Whether you believe in the secular scientists' view that the theory of evolution is correct, or you believe that we were a divine creation of God, the fundamental answers are still the same regarding metabolic types.

I spend time on this only because I do not want anyone to waste time or energy thinking that anything I have written conflicts with their belief systems. It is also my habit to present balance in arguments as much as I can. Then it is up to the reader to use the objective information I have provided to improve their health.

The book of Genesis (followed by Hebrews, Christians and Muslims), clearly tells us that all foods were provided in the Garden of Eden, but God didn't serve up meals to Adam and Eve on a silver platter; they still had to gather their food. There are passages in Genesis that could be interpreted to support the case for vegetarianism or an omnivorous diet. I am working on a separate book that objectively covers that controversy, but it would simply take too much space to address the issue here and it would not affect our decisions on metabolic typing. My purpose here is simply to say that in the beginning, regardless of your belief systems, our earliest ancestors were not farmers and were not designed to eat refined foods. That last thought has an absolute effect on finding your metabolic type.

The book of Genesis tells us that in the beginning God created the perfect garden and placed Adam in it.

2:8 And the LORD God planted a garden eastward in Eden; and there He put the man whom He had formed.

*2:9 And out of the ground made the LORD God to grow **every tree that is pleasant to the sight, and good for food**; the tree of life also in the midst of the garden, and the tree of knowledge of good and evil.*

Once Adam and Eve were expelled from the Garden of Eden, they had to work for their food; they began farming and herding. There is no indication that they had begun farming before being expelled from the garden.

*3:17 And unto Adam He said, Because thou hast hearkened unto the voice of thy wife, and hast eaten of the tree, of which I commanded thee, saying, Thou shalt not eat of it**: cursed [is] the ground for thy sake; in sorrow shalt thou eat [of] it all the days of thy life;***

*3:18 **Thorns also and thistles shall it bring forth to thee; and thou shalt eat the herb of the field;***

*3:19 **In the sweat of thy face shalt thou eat bread, till thou return unto the ground**; for out of it was thou taken: for dust thou [art], and unto dust shalt thou return.*

*3:23 **Therefore the LORD God sent him forth from the Garden of Eden, to till the ground from whence he was taken.***

When Europeans first colonized America they called the natives they encountered Indians because they had mistakenly believed they had sailed around the world and landed in India. Most of the "American Indians" they found were Stone Age people, not having discovered even the most rudimentary metals. Most of the native tribes in North America were quintessential hunter-gatherers; there were a few notable exceptions that had rudimentary farming but relied significantly on hunting as well. Without belaboring the point there were some Native American cultures that were Stone Age farmers, but that discussion is lengthy and detracts from the point of this discussion.

The point is that in the beginning all our ancestors were Stone Age people. There are only a few rare examples of these primitive peoples still in existence today. We call them hunter-gatherers because they are nomadic and have no real cultural or scientific achievements. They have to spend most of every day hunting and gathering food. A few of these peoples influenced by us today have a mix of hunter-gatherer behavior with some of our technologies such as the Inuit of the Arctic Circle.

Each of these groups has adapted over time to the food available in their environment and to the environment itself.

For example, the Inuit people (incorrectly called Eskimos by many Americans,) must eat a diet high in fat and protein to be healthy. This adaptation occurred because the only foods available from their environment are highly fatty animals and fish. There are no grains, vegetables, or fruits. So the Inuit consume a high-protein/high-fat diet, but remain free of heart disease and hypertension, as long as they do not mix high G foods from our modern diet with the foods they were adapted to eat. Raw animal or fish protein provides everything they need, nutrient wise.

Science has also shown that the colder it is the more fat you burn, because fat is where our energy calories are stored and the colder it is the more energy you need to maintain your core body temperature. This is another reason that the Inuit, who live in the Arctic Circle, need to eat more fat. The assumption that they have no heart disease is because they get Omega three essential fatty acids from fish is a good marketing story, but in reality only a contributing factor, not the whole story. Omega three's are indeed essential to life and do in fact help to breakdown fat in your body, however, it has taken centuries of adaptation for the Inuit to be able to eat so much fat and stay healthy.

Another excellent example are the Pima Indians of the U.S. state of New

Mexico and the nation of Mexico. They are genetically the same group separated by an artificial political boundary. Those in the U.S. are now the fattest population in the United States. However, their genetically identical counterparts in Mexico are lean. The U.S. group suffers from virtually every health problem that relates to fat—including diabetes, heart disease, hypertension and stroke—while the group in Mexico are virtually free of these problems. Why? Because the U.S. Pima Indians eat the modern U.S. low fat but high-glycemic diet. Their cousins in Mexico still eat the traditional, low-glycemic ancestral diet.

Another scientific example can be made regarding near-sightedness and high G foods. Humans, living in the original environmental niche for which our species is genetically adapted (as hunter-gatherers), are either slightly hypermetropic or emmetropic and rarely develop myopia.[18] The word hypermetropic is from Latin, but originally taken from the Greek huper (later hyper) beyond and metros meaning measure. This is an adjective to describe hyperopia or far-sightedness. Emmetropic is also taken from Greek. Ops means eye and emmetros a derivative of Greek metron (measure) and interpreted as normal measure.

Myopia (near-sightedness) occurs when novel environmental conditions associated with modern civilization are introduced into the hunter-gatherer lifestyle.[18] Remember I talked about the fact that some hunter-gatherers, like the Inuit, have been influenced by us and therefore, are not true hunter-gatherers anymore and are now suffering with "modern illnesses" as we are.

Excessive amounts of close-up work, such as reading, is most frequently cited as the main environmental stressor underlying the development of myopia by most researchers. However, in a recent study a diet-related malady (chronic hyperinsulinemia) was mentioned and may play a key role in the pathogenesis of juvenile-onset myopia because of its interaction with hormonal regulation of vitreal chamber growth.[18] The vitreous chamber is between the lens and the back of the eye, derived from the Latin vitrium meaning glass. I was one of those children who developed severe juvenile myopia, because of entirely high G diet due to financial constraints.

This is just another of many new studies supporting the theory that it is our departure from the diet we were genetically predetermined to eat, that is causing many of our health issues today. Additionally, this also supports the idea that high glycemic foods, which cause hyperinsulin responses, are bad for everyone, whether there is weight gain or not.

The Masai tribesmen of Africa eat a diet almost exclusively composed of animal protein and fat. They have one of the lowest known incidences of heart disease, obesity and hypertension. Why? Because they are genetically adapted to their environment, and giving them foods they are not adapted to would have disastrous consequences for their health.

Their greatest resource is cattle. It is not only a symbol of wealth for them it is also the basis of their diet. They let blood from the cattle and mix it with milk from the cows, then twirl it on a stick while it dries in the hot sun and it becomes a sort of all day protein sucker. They try not to eat too many of the animals because that diminishes their wealth as well as reduces their potential food supply. That milk and blood, which you may find distasteful, provides huge nutrition, not just protein and fat (for calories), but vitamins and minerals as well. We shouldn't judge other cultures by our standards. Whether you like it or not, it has worked well for them for centuries.

The Masai and Inuit (like the Pima Indians of New Mexico) will get heart disease fast if given low fat but high glycemic foods. At the same time, genetic types that have adapted over time to a lower protein or lower fat diet will suffer quickly if put on the Inuit diet.

The diet best for you will make you likely to achieve and maintain healthy body composition, as well as optimal health.

There are many factors involved in metabolic typing and in human adaptation. I will not attempt to discuss each in detail, but I will give an overview for the absolutists who are looking for a reason not to succeed on this or any other diet.

The earliest attempts at metabolic typing date back many decades. These were done primarily by observation without the benefit of the scientific method. Later, studies were conducted to find a correlation between disease and diet. Many years ago I was inspired by the work of the late Dr. Roger Williams, which set me on the path of metabolic individuality.[18] It was his work that motivated me to do postgraduate study in biological anthropology and sparked my interest in human adaptation to diet and environment.

There have been many methods published since Williams and there is no point in discussing them all. One that deserves mention is a book by a Naturopathic doctor named P.J. D'Adamo, titled Eat Right For Your Type. It is very popular with lay audiences due to his ingenious simplification of a very complex topic, and the bottom line is that the laymen are the population seeking wellness. The medical community, with few exceptions, are still not willing to look beyond low fat or low cal. D'Adamo's book is based on an evolutionary principal that each blood type evolved over time and has a unique set of food requirements.

Dr. D'Adamo's book makes a plausible analysis of blood types and the best diet for each blood type. Without actually doing a long-term controlled study, I would say based on my observations of patients over the years, that his book gives some very good guidelines and insights, but as is the case with every metabolic typing method including serum analysis (which is by far the most accurate), there are exceptions. This may be due to a wide variety of factors including some not yet discovered. Most medical doctors, by virtue of their training, are unwilling to consider his theory.

For decades I have stated in my lectures, everyone is biochemically and genetically unique. All doctors who care about their patients success are trying to find the most effective, yet easy to understand, ways of explaining and guiding people to success with their health. The current state of science in this area has not yet revealed all we need to know to be 100% accurate in all cases with any method or theory.

Body morphology typing is commonly used by many laymen because you can do it at a glance and no lab testing is required. Later you see it corresponds (graphically) with nervous system typing.

Serum Analysis, Blood testing not Blood Typing
Since this book is designed to help the average person, not to train doctors necessarily, I will be very brief regarding lab tests. Also any health care practitioner can take the Category One Continuing Medical Education training I do on metabolic typing and glycemic indexing for healthy body composition, if they want the technical information.

Serum analysis represents a more quantifiable method however…a review of 74 papers showed there was still inconsistency in this testing method.[19] With the potential variables, it is unlikely with current technology that a 100% reliable test will be found. Ask your physician to run the blood tests and interpret them for you.

With serum analysis, most practitioners use five types. Some divide further into more subtypes but the subtypes serve no purpose with diet recommendation; I will not discuss those here. The five basic types are sometimes also referred to as Phenotypes and sometimes referred to as categories of Hyperlipoproteinemia.[16]

Hyperlipoproteinemia is a scary word. It refers to any of several disorders of lipoprotein and cholesterol metabolism that result in high levels of lipoprotein and cholesterol in the blood. Hyper is high, lipoprotien refers to a biochemical mixture of fat and protein. When there are elevated levels of lipoprotiens in the blood cholesterol levels are also high, which leads to increased risk of heart and blood vessel disease. Ok. Let's move on. Regardless of the label used by a given lab for the test, you are still looking for the same things and for the same reasons. Although abnormalities in Types I, II and III can give information about the potential for heart disease or diabetes, in these types it is not significantly useful in terms of weight loss. So, I have divided the five types into two groups.

Simplified for weight loss in two groups
•Group 1
–Type I, II, III
•Group 2
–Type IV, V
Only type IV and V will need weight loss for health reasons and this is not meant to be a textbook.

Hyperlipoproteinemia or Pheno ype IV Characteristics
   •Corresponds to Type GK4
   •Thrifty gene
   •Varying degrees of carbohydrate sensitivity
   •Varying degrees of insulin resistance
   •Males central obesity
   •Females (pear shaped) typically thighs and buttocks
   •Corresponds to Parasympathetic dominant
   •Typically blood type O or B
   •Corresponds to Metabolic Syndrome, also known as Syndrome X
      or insulin resistant
   •The degree of insulin resistance varies between patients but the dietary
      recommendations are still low glycemic.

Most common type with
   •Obesity
   •Diabetes
   •Pre-diabetics
   •Atherosclerosis
   •Pre-Atherosclerosis
   •Highly sensitive to refined carbohydrates
   •Frequently insulin resistant

The blood tests show
- Triglycerides always elevated (although sometimes only slightly)
- Cholesterol normal or elevated
- Quantitatively the triglycerides always higher than cholesterol in Type IV's regardless
- Pre-Beta elevated above Beta region

This is genetic but the readings may appear in patients without this genetic disorder secondary to [16]
- Other metabolic disorders
- Psychological stress
- Excessive carbohydrate intake
- Excessive alcohol intake
- These readings always exacerbated by obesity

This is why even serum analysis is not 100% accurate.

They process fats more efficiently than other types, so low fat diets are least effective on Type IV's. They are the least capable of all types of processing carbohydrates, so they tend to initially do the best on low carb diet. Low carb is a long-term mistake with Type IV's, the "Thrifty Gene" will cause adaptation.

Whether a true genetic Type IV or not the same steps are recommended.
- Low glycemic foods only!
- Restrict alcohol intake
- Progressive exercise program, begin with caution
- Type IV's have the "Thrifty Gene" so portions should be small with grazing recommended
- The Type IV is still a hunter-gather whether they like it or not.

Hyperlipoproteinemia Type V was a type IV for at least 10 years prior to the onset of adult diabetes. Same information applies but it is far more risky for a Type V to eat high glycemic foods. Type V's always correspond to GK5.

One method of lab testing almost never used is to request a serum (blood) protein electrophoresis or SPE. I haven't seen any doctors I know request that one for more than 10 years, but I'll mention it anyway. Blood is drawn and a graph is compiled from the results. The doctor then has to know which sections of the graph represent each category of proteins and fats and know what peaks and valleys in each mean. It is laborious and complicated. The average clinical practitioner doesn't have the time or the inclination for this sort of thing.

The Simple Answer
Regardless of theory or method of arriving at Type, no high G foods are allowed for anyone who wants to be healthy. My rules for getting into the GK Zone will show you the easy way to do this. Moderate exercise at least every other day progressing with appropriate levels of fitness for Type IV and V, but not until after your doctor has given you the go ahead. Serum analysis is the most accurate but patients who need "real" help with weight loss will always present as Type IV's or Type V's, which always correspond, to GK 4 or GK5 that you are going to learn about.

You can do this at home kids

Your nervous system and your metabolism
Last, I will discuss a method you can do yourself, without labs or complicated math; it is based on the nervous system theory. Please take the time to patiently read this information before you take your Genetic Key Survey.

The nervous system plays a significant role in forming your physical and emotional make-up. It determines how you will react to various events and conditions, regardless of other factors. Genetics sets the stage for virtually everything.

Understanding the Nervous system
Before I start this section understand that some people want more technical data and some do not. If you think some of the next few paragraphs are too complicated for you, don't worry, I will make it <u>very</u> simple afterwards.

Your nervous system has two major divisions—the central nervous system (CNS) and the peripheral nervous system. The central nervous system contains the spinal cord and the brain.

The peripheral nervous system has two parts—the somatic and autonomic nervous systems. The somatic consists of nerves that convey messages from the sense organs to the CNS and then to the muscles and glands. The autonomic nervous system is a set of neurons controlling the heart, intestines, and other organs.

The autonomic nervous system also has two parts—the sympathetic and parasympathetic; that's where metabolism comes in. The sympathetic has two paired chains of ganglia (collections of neuron cell bodies). Axons extend from the sympathetic nervous system to the organs.

The sympathetic system prepares the body for "fight or flight," increases heart and breathing rates, and decreases digestive activity. Since all sympathetic ganglia are linked, they act together—"in sympathy" with one another.

The parasympathetic nervous system has functions related to, but generally opposite from, those of the sympathetic system. Although these systems oppose each other, they usually act simultaneously. However, the balance of activity may sometimes tilt more toward one system or the other, resulting in one side dominating the other, temporarily or continuously, in some individuals.

Parasympathetic activity decreases heart rate, increases digestive rate, may cause more frequency of bowel activity for some and generally promotes energy-conserving, non-emergency functions. Energy conservation means slow fat burn but efficient fat storage (the Thrifty Gene concept), making consistently parasympathetic people more prone to illness and weight problems.

The role of food
Choosing the right food is important for your overall health and weight management. Anyone familiar with my lectures for laymen or my Category One Continuing Medical Education seminars on weight management probably knows that I always recommend a low-glycemic or low moderate glycemic diet for everyone. Even for people who don't need to lose weight. Other diets are proven failures. Low-glycemic foods do not trigger the undesirable insulin reaction that shuts down the normal process by which the body converts fat as energy. No matter your metabolic type or blood type, the benefits of a low G diet are simply too powerful to ignore.

Every person should clearly understand the role of fats and proteins. Proteins provide the basic building blocks of life, called *amino acids*. Without these, you could not exist. Animal proteins are very high in amino acids, vitamins and minerals because herbivores (exclusive plant eaters) that are the source for the meats people eat are designed to get all the nutrients they need from vegetable or plant matter, and then store it in their muscles.

Dairy associations have done a superb job of convincing everyone that calcium only comes from milk or milk products. That's simply not the case. Herbivore muscle tissue, which we refer to collectively as "meat," is high in calcium and other vital minerals because muscles can't function without calcium, magnesium, potassium, and phosphorus, as well as B vitamins. Meat contains B_{12} which explains why many human vegetarians frequently become B_{12} deficient. Without calcium, you will not only have weak bones, but also muscle cramps.

Since herbivorous animals must eat most of the day they can't afford to have muscle cramps, which will surely occur without the above-mentioned minerals.

Humans who eat low-nutritive diets must eat far more food than other people, and must eat constantly, like cows. They tend to become very large. This is a lesson from nature to make sure that we get a widely varied and balanced diet, as well as maximum nutritional support.

Despite what some non-science authors have portrayed in vegetarian literature, humans do not have the same or even similar digestive systems as those in herbivores (exclusive plant eaters), nor do we have the systems of carnivores (exclusive meat eaters). We are omnivores. That word is from the Latin *Omni* meaning all and *vores* meaning to eat. The human digestive system is designed to digest both plant and animal material, explaining why humans are neither herbivores nor carnivores. Different types need different amounts and proportions of animal and vegetable, as you will soon find out.

Some vegetables contain proteins, as do grains, nuts, and seeds. Vegetables alone, however, must be properly combined for you to derive the protein value you need since no individual vegetable provides complete protein amino acid balance. The human body requires proteins to maintain healthy muscle mass and continuous energy, as well as normal blood sugar.

How to interpret your GKS results

The score of your GKS will place you in one of five general body type categories. These categories and their dietary recommendations are summarized here and explained more fully in the GKS. You can answer the questions on the GKS and find out your type now or later, but either way you need to have an explanation of the types.

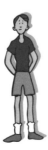

GK1 leans more towards sympathetic function than balanced function. The

sympathetic nervous system prepares the body for "fight or flight" activities. It increases the heart rate and breathing rate and decreases digestive activity. Since all sympathetic ganglia are closely linked, they tend to act as a single system. They act "in sympathy" with one another, hence the name. Their blood type is likely to be A or AB, but due to centuries of contact between various genetic groups, blood type is no longer fully predictable. I have seen type GK1 patients who were type blood B or O, but matched all parameters for the type GK1.

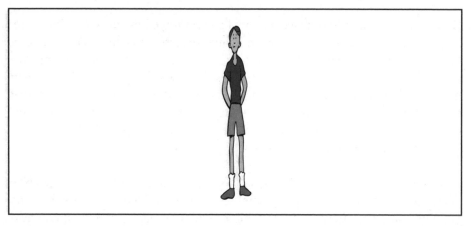

GK2 is highly sympathetic dominant and typically would be naturally thin and tall as compared to your other family members, not just as compared to the general population. Often, but not always, the GK 2 will typically look older than they are. Their metabolism is faster and that, of course, accelerates the aging process. They would be the type of person who never seems to gain weight, even when they eat high fat or high G foods.

A GK2 metabolism would run high, possibly having a tendency to constipation and thriving (without weight gain) on a diet high in carbohydrates. Their blood type is likely to be AB or A, but due to centuries of contact between various genetic groups, blood type is no longer fully predictable. I have occasionally seen type GK1 patients who were blood type B or O, but matched all parameters for the type GK2.

GK1's and GK2's have the lowest need and generally the lowest desire for protein from the three basic groups. They are the only body type that can be healthy on a properly designed vegetarian diet. The emphasis is on "properly designed." Too many individuals who wish to become vegetarians for philosophical or religious reasons are not genetically suited for that lifestyle and do so without proper education in this area. This approach can result in less than optimal health. Indeed, I had many sick vegetarians come to my clinic for help.

GK1 and GK2 can do very well as a vegetarian. It is important that they learn how to combine vegetable protein properly to be healthy. The person with predominant **GK1** or GK2 traits is often less efficient in producing protein-digesting enzymes, often has digestive difficulties, and can usually benefit from taking digestive enzyme supplements. They may also find that if they do not cook their vegetables that digestive enzymes are essential. They also frequently must take hydrochloric acid supplements when consuming animal protein since they tend to be more alkaline in general. They may complain that they do not like meat or that meat makes them feel uncomfortable.

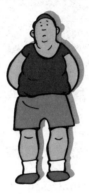

GK 4 leans more towards parasympathetic function than balanced function. This type generally digests protein and conserves energy well—a pronounced advantage in times of famine, but a real problem in modern countries where food is too easily available. Their diets need to be lower in carbohydrates because they tend to gain weight quickly due to their energy conservation capacity.[17] This type is more prone to illness, blood sugar abnormalities, fatigue, weight gain, and other adverse health conditions.

GK 4 actually needs animal proteins in some way to receive the complete spectrum of amino acids, vitamins, and minerals to be well. All things being equal, they digest heavy proteins efficiently but are very inefficient at converting most carbohydrates as energy. When type GK4 or GK5's attempt to become vegetarians they are always overweight, despite the fact they avoid fats and animal protein.

The ancient conservation mechanism I have discussed in this book turns carbohydrates into stored fat and blood fats just in case there is a food shortage. We do not need that mechanism in the modern world today but the body doesn't know this. These types simply cannot tolerate high G foods and although they may be psychologically determined to be vegetarians, it simply doesn't work for their physiology.

Because the GK 4 and GK5 are not well suited to subsist on carbohydrates alone, and since they are more prone to drops in blood sugar than the other types, they tend never to be satisfied by carbohydrates—especially of the high-glycemic variety—and as a result, their appetite for those carbohydrates is often unceasing. I strongly recommend that they always eat low G or they will be very unlikely to stay in the GK Zone.

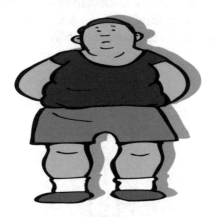

GK 4 and GK 5's represent the quintessential hunter-gatherer. Our hunter-gatherer ancestors, as well as the few hunter-gatherer tribes still left today were and are food generalists who ate whatever they could find. They were constantly on the move and had the ability to conserve energy efficiently. They usually ate an average of 5 to 6 small meals per day.[18,19] The ancient food conservation mechanism is most efficient in this type which makes them most likely to be obese in the modern world, by consuming high G foods.

Usually, GK 4's and GK 5's have a soft body, low energy, and hold weight around the waist and face for men, and from the waist down for women (pear shape). A diet high in high G carbohydrates will cause male or female GK 4's to put on weight at virtually any point of the body (apple shape).

This type needs more B vitamins to produce all digestive enzymes, maintain blood sugar control, and energy. Their requirement for antioxidant support is lower than that of the GK1, 2, or 3, but their need for blood sugar and metabolic support is higher than other types. So they should have chromium, and vanadium in daily supplements and most of them will also benefit from iodine as well. That is a general statement and a specific analysis would be required to be completely accurate.

GK 5's are very poorly suited for vegetarianism. GK 4's who are only slightly parasympathetic-dominant are better suited as long as they have proper educa-tion.

GK 3's are balanced types in nearly every way. In general, they can eat and digest the complete range of foods available to humans from all food groups with relative efficiency. They comprise the majority of a <u>healthy</u> population because the nervous system of a healthy individual is designed to work in bal-ance.

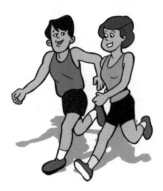

GK 3's should consume approximately 3-4 ounces of protein at least twice daily, or as often as three times daily, if they are very active (as most B's are). If GK 3 is doing an <u>extraordinary level</u> of resistance training, they may need to use more than 100 grams of protein daily for males and 75 grams for females. This type is the truly balanced omnivore and is poorly suited for vegetarian diets.

Regarding protein servings: I recommend the very popular palm of the hand rule as it is simple and most often is very accurate. Each of us has a different size palm and it corresponds with our body size. When I mention this in a lecture there is always someone looking for a reason to cheat, (which ends up cheating no one but themselves), and they will ask, "Just how thick is that piece of meat that sits in my palm?" Use common sense. A grilled chicken breast will fit in most adult palms; it is not very thick is it? The other aspect of measure is weight. Do not eat more than 6 ounces of animal protein at a single sitting. Heavy pro-teins are difficult to digest, so to do it efficiently, eat small portions frequently rather than a 24 ounces T Bone steak in a single sitting. Bigger isn't better in this case and "all you can eat" is not a bargain for your health!

Even though they can eat from all groups, and weight management is often not a severe problem, GK 3's should still avoid all high-G carbohydrates. They will, however, do well with moderate and low-G carbohydrates.

In today's environment, this body type requires a balanced vitamin/mineral formula with good antioxidant support, but they have no unusual need for additional blood sugar or metabolic support. Unless specifically diagnosed with a deficiency of vitamins or minerals, this type should only be taking a daily vitamin mineral supplement. All types, however, in today's environment, need to be taking an antioxidant and glyconutrient supplement daily.[24,25,26] That is the subject of two other books I have written.

Ok, now take the brief survey, and let's find out your Genetic Key.

Genetic Key Survey (GKS)

Directions:

Check only one box in each of the four columns.

Check the box that most closely applies to you the majority of the time.

There are no right or wrong, good or bad answers, and you do not need to show your score to anyone else. To get the most accurate results, please make sure you are as candid and honest as possible in your responses.

Don't "overthink" your answers.

Take as much time as you need and read all statements carefully since they are carefully worded, and some may look very similar.

If none of the first three boxes in any row apply to you, check the fourth box in that row.

When you have finished, please follow the directions to total your score.

Please consider completing this survey with a friend or loved one who knows you best. You'll have fun learning more about yourself and you're sure to get the most objective results.

Physical	Physical	Physical	
COLUMN 1	COLUMN 2	COLUMN 3	COLUMN 4
1. My energy levels are normally high	My energy levels are normally low, and I need to use things like caffeine or something similar to give me enough energy to keep up the pace I need.	My energy levels are about the same as everyone else's.	
2. Humidity doesn't bother me much, and I prefer hot weather to cold.	Humidity really bothers me, and I prefer cool weather to hot.	I adapt easily to temperature changes.	
3. My blood pressure is high without using medication	My blood pressure is low to normal without using medication.	My blood pressure is normal without using medication.	I don't know how my blood pressure runs.
4. My body temperature runs normal, but I *often* feel cold when others are warm.	My body temperature typically runs slightly below normal and I *may* feel cold when others are warm.	My body temperature is always normal unless I get sick, and I always feel comfortably warm.	
5. Eating beef can upset my stomach.	Raw vegetables give me gas.		
6. I don't like salty foods.	If I could eat any snacks I want without regard to weight gain or health issues, I would often choose salty snacks like chips or popcorn.	I really have no preference.	
7. I have no allergies or allergic symptoms that I know of.	I have seasonal allergies. These may be minor or major, chronic or periodic		
8. I have excellent stamina and can keep going longer than the average person.	I have average to below-average stamina unless I supplement my diet to keep up my endurance.	I have average stamina.	

9. I have thick or hard fingernails.	I have thin or weak fingernails.		
10. If I get sick at all, I usually recover more quickly than most people.	I have had illnesses like head colds or flu that took more than 10 days to get over.	It *never* takes me more than 10 days to recover from illnesses like colds and flu.	
11. I require very little sleep. I can do well on less than 6 hours per night.	I need my sleep. I need 7 or even more hours per night to feel good the next day.		
12. I have normal to high blood sugar without using medication.	I have low to normal blood sugar. *Or* I have occasional hypoglycemic symptoms between meals.	I have normal blood sugar without using medication.	I don't know my blood sugar levels between meals.
13. If I could have any dessert I want without regard to weight gain or health issues, I would choose something sweet but not rich or fatty.	If I could have any dessert I want without regard to weight gain or health issues, I would often choose rich desserts.		
14. I rarely am tired.	I feel tired in the afternoon between 1-5 pm unless I use caffeine or something similar for an energy boost.	I don't feel tired until bedtime.	
15. I sometimes have difficulty getting to sleep, but not staying asleep.	I have no difficulty getting to sleep, but sometimes have difficulty staying asleep.	I have no difficulty getting to sleep or staying asleep.	
16. I feel sluggish or even sleepy after eating meat.	When I first eat a carbohydrate food, I feel good, but I may feel sluggish or even sleepy 20 to 30 minutes after eating carbohydrates—especially refined carbohydrates.	I don't feel sluggish or sleepy after eating either carbohydrates or proteins.	
17. I am *never* hungry between meals.	I am *sometimes* hungry between meals.		
18. I rarely have mood swings, but if I have a change in mood, it is typically normal to high.	If I have mood swings, they tend to be more down than up. *Or* I have frequent mood swings.	I rarely have mood swings in any direction.	
19. I feel full with small amounts of food.	It seems I have to eat a lot before I feel satisfied or full. *Or* there are certain foods that I can't seem to get enough of.		
20. I sometimes feel jittery if I use caffeine.	I really need my morning coffee or tea.	Coffee doesn't make me jittery, and I don't need coffee or tea in the morning.	
21. I have consistent energy even if I miss meals.	I feel tired and sometimes even cranky if I miss meals.		
22. I am consistently mentally alert all day.	I have decreased mental alertness in the afternoons unless I eat or drink something that perks me up, such as coffee, tea, cola, candy or pastry.		
23. I am over 6 ft. tall if male, or over 5' 5" tall if female.	I am 6 ft. tall or less if male, or 5' 5" tall or less if female.		
24. I don't have to lose weight. Most people consider me slim.	I have a constant problem since I always carry extra weight. *And/or* I have difficulty losing weight and keeping it off	I don't have a real weight problem, but if I need to lose weight, it is not very difficult getting it off fast.	

25. Most of my family members appear to be thinner than the average for North Americans.	Many of my family members are more than 10 pounds over-weight or even have serious weight problems.	Most males in my family have a waistline that is not more than 40 inches, and most females in my family have a waistline that is not more than 35 inches	
26. I have no trouble with weight retention.	I tend to retain weight in my hips and thighs (if female), or waist (if male)	When I retain weight, it tends to be very slight and about evenly distributed throughout my body	
27. Even the smell of cooking meat bothers me.	I enjoy meats. I couldn't imagine meals without them.	I eat meat occasionally, but I can do without it	
28. I like sweet tastes, but chocolate is too rich for me.	I really enjoy chocolate and it's rich, creamy textures. Eating chocolate can sometimes make me feel better psychologically too.	I do like the taste of chocolate, but I can take it or leave it. It doesn't affect my emotions that I am aware of.	
29. I prefer breads and pastas to meats.	I think a meal with meat is not complete without breads or pastas.	I enjoy some breads and pastas, but having a meal without them is okay.	
30. I can make a meal out of a loaded baked potato without meat.	Whenever I have a meal with meat, it doesn't feel complete unless I have a potato in some form.	I like potatoes but can do without them.	
31. I can eat Chinese food and feel satisfied for hours.	When I eat Chinese food, I always get hungry again with in an hour.		
32. My favorite breakfast would be fruits and/or cereals, and maybe pastry.	If I could have any breakfast I want without regard to weight gain or health issues, I would definitely choose eggs with meat and bread in some form.	If I could have any breakfast I want without regard to weight gain or health issues, I would definitely choose pastries, doughnuts or cereals.	
33 I think I appear older than my actual age.	I think I appear younger than my actual age.	I think I look my age.	
34. I have a tendency to dry skin.	I have a tendency to oily and/or supple skin.	I have average skin.	
35. I can eat any amount or type of carbohydrate and not gain weight.	I must eat little or no carbohydrates to keep from gaining weight.	I can eat some carbohydrates and not gain weight.	
36. I can eat any carbohydrate and still lose weight.	I must eat very limited amounts or even no carbohdrates in order to lose weight.	I can lose weight eating anything, as long as I reduce the amounts I eat.	
37. I may go a day or more without having a bowel movement.	I often have three or more bowel movements in a day.	I have one to three bowel movements daily.	
38. I love to exercise. Or I just need to be active.	I don't like exercise because it's work.	Exercise feels good when I do it, but if I miss it, it doesn't break my heart.	
39. I never feel light-headed if I stand up quickly after sitting or lying down for a few minutes.	If I stand up quickly after sitting or lying down for a few minutes, I sometimes feel light-headed.	I rarely feel lightheaded for any reason.	
40. I have lost weight easier in the past by avoiding fats.	I have lost weight easier in the past with low-carbohydrate diets.	I have lost weight easier in the past with low-calorie diets.	I have never dieted, or I have never used those diets in. columns 1, 2, or 3.

Please enter the total number of boxes you checked in Column 1.	Please enter the total number of boxes you checked in Column 2.	Please enter the total number of boxes you checked in Column 3.
If you scored the highest number in this column, you are a **Type GK1**	If you scored the highest number in this column, you are a **Type GK4**	If you scored the highest number in this column, you are a **Type GK3**
If you checked 25 or more boxes in this column, you are a **Type GK2**	If you checked 25 or more boxes in this column, you are a **Type GK5**	*Note:* There are fewer choices in this **GK3** column because we are now attempting to ascertain two types.

NOTE: It would be rare to find someone who represented 100% of the traits of one type—because we are all genetically and biochemically unique. Even within a family that has the same genetic parents, offspring has differently colored eyes, hair, skin and even blood types from one of their parents and their siblings. It is not unusual for someone to be one type physically and another type psychologically. With this in mind, this survey is designed only to give you some basic direction in both diet selection and choosing your daily supplements.

The ideal state of the nervous system is a state of balance. However, because of genes, lifestyle choices and other factors, not everyone achieves that ideal state.

It is not uncommon for someone to be dominant on one side of the nervous system. People with similar nervous systems often share many physical and behavioral traits. Below are some examples of common characteristics often seen in people with sympathetic and parasympathetic body types.

Below are some examples of behavioral traits sometimes seen with each type, however, I would caution that there are many factors that influence behavior, so please use the physical characteristics on the GKS, not these traits to arrive at your Genetic Key.

GK 1 Intellectually bright, tends to be impatient, cool but perceives him/herself as warm, and no one can convince them otherwise. They are caring, efficient, organized, and tend to dominate conversations or meetings.

GK 2 Tends to be a type A emotionally as well as blood type A or AB, there are of course exceptions. Once again, there are exceptions because many factors affect behavior and even unwanted behaviors can be changed. A person with a type A personality can learn to be more calm and relaxed if they first can see themselves realistically and second, if they have a genuine desire to change. Life is full of choices.

GK 4 very friendly, thoughtful and thorough, very patient, listens well, passionate and perceived by virtually everyone as warm, caring, trustworthy, a little disorganized, and quiet until they have something to contribute to a discussion.

GK 5 too open about their own feelings, lethargic, rarely completes anything, often feels victimized, often mentally unfocused, frequently depressed, often dependent on others, untidy about virtually everything, but will say they know where something is in a pile. They may be reluctant to join in conversations unless they are confident they have the answer and, at that point, it may be difficult to get them to stop talking.

The GK 4 AND 5'S share so many traits that they often have some of both categories in terms of traits. Remember behavior is influenced by many factors, genetics is only one of them.

Simple Summary of the Genetic Key (GK types)

GK 4 and 5
- •Oldest Genetic Type
- •Parasympathetic dominant
- •Lower metabolic rate
- •The Thrifty Gene*
- •Thrives on protein
- •Becomes obese with refined carbs
- •Often hypothyroid
- •Corresponds with serum analysis type IV and V
- •Often, but not always blood type O or B
- •Omnivore; fresh raw natural diet required for optimal health.
- •Low end of normal to normal on thyroid and TSH (thyroid stimulating hormone)
- •Greater incidence of, obesity, heart disease, and diabetes than the other GK types

GK 1 and GK 2
- •Sympathetic dominant
- •Tolerates carbs better-tends not to store hanging fat
- •Naturally thin
- •Normal to hyperthyroid.
- •Newest type thrives on carbs
- •High end of normal on TSH and Thyroid panel
- •Sometimes hyperthyroid
- •Often, but not always, blood type A or AB
- •Up to 15% taller than average*
- •Still may fall victim to heart disease and diabetes if they consume high G foods

The GENETIC KEY Diet

SECTION 4

Appetite plateaus and nutrition

The Key to Unlock a Lean Body & a Long Healthy Life

by Dr. Steve Nugent

Chapter 6
What's the reason for increased appetite and how do you control it?

As research continues, we will no doubt continue to have new information on appetite control. In February 2006, some new data on appetite control, as it relates to hormones, was published. Before I get to that new information, let's look at the three primary reasons for increased appetite that we can do something about.

1. A drop in blood sugar
    a. Hormonal signals
2. A need for nutrients
    a. Hormonal signals
3. Feeling of Fullness

There are two other minor factors: Psychological stimuli and Sleep; I will discuss them shortly, but for now, let's address the big three.

How do nutritional supplements help you to control your appetite?
If your body is low on a given nutrient, your brain will make you crave foods that it knows contain that nutrient. So, taking at the minimum, a complete vitamin mineral supplement everyday is essential to your success. If you are a slow metabolic type, all the more reason to take a multivitamin designed for the purpose of supporting metabolism.

Keeping your blood sugar normal is absolutely essential to your success. So, not only do you need to take a dietary supplement that is at least the minimum of chromium and B complex, but you should also supplement vanadium, which is important to pancreatic function. Note that in some countries vanadium (a trace mineral) is unknown to the regulators so the result is it is not permitted in those countries. In many countries regulators are MD's or trained in the allopathic method and do not recognize any value in even common supplements, let alone cutting edge supplementation. Vanadium gives you a slight edge for pancreatic health and function, but chromium and B complex are key.

Feeling full
There are receptors in the stomach that tell the brain when you are full. When they have pressure against them you "feel full" and for some people this is adequate most of the time. Some people will engorge themselves in an attempt to

accomplish this feeling. Most people I have observed use their flatware like a shovel. They are in some sort of a desperate race to shovel as much volume as they can into their mouths as quickly as possible. Most people do this without realizing it. Stress, and the hectic pace of modern life, as well as short lunch hours, tend to contribute to this phenomenon. You need to put that fork down on the table (out of your hand) in between bites. Chew your food thoroughly, it's your first step to success.

I recommend either a glucomannan or a pectin fiber supplement to help reduce your appetite. When taken with 8 ounces of filtered H_2O, they gently expand against those receptors in your stomach.

Glucomannan is high in fiber, essential for cleaning the digestive system. Glucomannan is taken from the Konnyaku root native to Japan (often called konjac) and is from the same family as the yam, and is 100 percent natural dietary fiber without calories. Since lack of fiber is a major cause for the high incidence of growing gastrointestinal disorders, it is a valuable herb.

It helps reduce cholesterol, helps maintain regularity and promotes bowel health. It helps to normalize blood sugar, to relieve stress on the pancreas and to discourage blood sugar abnormalities, such as hypoglycemia (low blood sugar).

Glucomannan absorbs toxic substances produced during digestion and elimination. It binds toxic material and eliminates them before they can be absorbed into the blood stream.

Glucomannan acts as a prevention of chronic disease and a weight control agent. As a diet aid, it gently expands to dozens of times its original volume when used with a large glass of water. This certainly helps you feel full if you have sufficient glucomannan and sufficient water. It also may assist the body with the following issues so its benefits are certainly greater than just feeling full.

- Atherosclerosis
- Hemorrhoids
- Constipation
- High blood pressure
- Diabetes (high blood sugar)
- Hypoglycemia (low blood sugar)
- Digestive problems
- Obesity
- Diverticular disease
- Pancreas (reduce stress)

Pectin is a natural fiber found in fruits and vegetables. The meat of an apple, for example, is mostly pectin. Pectin is one of two nutritional reasons that apples are so good for you. Remember that old rhyme "An apple a day keeps the doctor away"?

Pectin fiber also assists the body with cleansing itself. Pectin can assist the body with:
- Removing daily toxins
- Removing heavy metals
- Removing damaged cellular material
- Lowering blood fats

Glucomannan is more efficient at achieving that feeling of fullness than pectin fiber, but pectin has unquestioned benefits. In some countries the regulators will not allow for glucomannan. They simply don't understand it and don't care to, so, in those countries pectin is the next best choice.

It is important to note that if your blood sugar is low, a feeling of fullness will not be enough to shut off the appetite. Eating too fast, as almost everyone I have observed does, will make things worse. It will take time for the food you eat to convert to a rise in blood sugar, especially if you eat low G foods, as you should. The faster you eat the more you will have to eat before the appetite receptors are satisfied. So… slow down!

Here is another important note on hormones. There are two hormones worth discussing, and in this short book I can't give either a complete explanation. The first one is called Cholecystikinin, or CCK for short. CCK can suppress the appetite and decrease the transit time of food as it passes through the gut, thus reducing calorie absorption.

CCK is released by the presence of fats in the duodenum, which is a sack below the stomach and the next place for digestion to occur. Its release rate is also increased by the presence of either L-isomer amino acids or calcium ions. So yes, calcium supplements can help to reduce appetite in some if taken about half an hour before food.

CCK increases the production of bile and bile salts and also causes contraction of the gall bladder and the bile duct. Bile salts aid the action of lipases by having a detergent like effect on fats. CCK also reduces appetite-there is a degree of controversy over this action. CCK is also produced in the brain, particularly in neurons innervating the lateral hypothalamus where the appetite centers are situated. It is not entirely clear whether CCK from the brain or the duodenum regulates food intake, possibly both. The main effect is to reduce food appetite, and therefore, food intake.

It takes time for fats to get into the duodenum, so once again, eating too fast will simply cause you to want to eat more. Eat slowly-enjoy the food. Try keeping it in your mouth long enough to enjoy the taste… now that's a novel concept.

In recent years, nutrition companies recognizing the studies on appetite and CCK, began promoting conjugated linoleic acids or CLA. CLA's do help to some extent (and have other benefits), but fish oil is far more efficient. The total range of health benefits from fish oil far outweighs the total benefits of CLA, and it is also more efficient at activating the CCK.

There is a patented molecular distillation process shown in third party university testing to remove chemicals from the fish oil but leaving its nutritional value intact. I will not recommend a brand, but I will say, that if the brand you are looking at doesn't clearly state they use this process, don't buy it! The chemicals, as well as mercury in untreated fish oils, can contribute to a wide variety of health issues from infertility to mental dysfunction to cancer.

Fish oils are technically called fats, but they are the so-called good fats also known as unsaturated fatty acids or EFA's. If you want proper hormone activity of any type, you better have your EFA's daily. You can't make them in your body, and although all animal products contain them, from fish to beef, cooking destroys most of the EFA's. So unless you are eating raw seafood daily, it is unlikely that you get enough in the modern diet. Warnings on excess seafood consumption has increased from 2004-2006. Fish is not the healthy value it used to be.[24,25] The average adult can benefit from at least 2400 mgs daily of supplements EFA's, however, many people need much more.

There are many hormones that we know of that effect appetite, but this is not a textbook on hormones. Since glucagon is discussed elsewhere I will only talk about one more hormone in this book.

It made the news in February 2006-it's called ghrelin. Ghrelin is a neurohormone (brain hormone), best known for its role in appetite and energy metabolism. That will make it a hit for the short spots on morning talk shows, but (less well-known) is the fact that it also influences learning and memory, according to a new study in *Nature Neuroscience*. A researcher, named Sabrino Diano of Yale University School of Medicine, along with her colleagues found that high levels of ghrelin in rodents could alter hippocampal (a part of the brain where memories are stored) morphology and improve performance on memory and learning tasks. Diano speculates that this pattern may provide an advantage, by boosting memory skills during food searches when animals are hungry. Another researcher, Robert Steiner of the University of Washington in Seattle, says it doesn't prove that normal levels of circulating ghrelin control learning and memory. Ghrelin is released primarily from stomach epithelial cells when the stomach is empty and binds to receptors in several areas of the body. It stimulates the release of growth hormone and also acts at hypothalamic feeding centers to increase hunger. Ghrelin receptors have also been found in many brain areas outside the hypothalamus including the hippocampus. The hypothalamus is your master gland and has the master control center for appetite as far as we know.[31,32,33,34,35,36,37,38,39,40,41,42,43,44,45]

This book isn't about memory, so let's get back to appetite. My greatest fear with ghrelin making the news, regarding appetite is that, many will misunderstand and misdirect the public. I fully expect those who do not understand the glycemic index and its crucial role in heart health, diabetes prevention, and achieving true fat loss, will recommend high glycemic foods to shut off that one appetite cause quickly. That is like throwing gasoline on a fire.

In fact, I saw one major morning talk show feature a dietitian recommending white potatoes to shut off ghrelin. First problem is that white potatoes are one of the worst things you can eat if you want to stay in the GK Zone, because they are very high G. So for many, this will present an adverse effect on blood sugar with all its consequences. Next, ghrelin is not the only factor in appetite control. In defense of the dietitian, those shows never allow anyone sufficient time to give a full explanation of any scientific subject and therefore often boost their ratings at the expense of full disclosure. In this case, it's a potential negative for many peoples' health.

Here is a better recommendation that is safe and will control ghrelin. Time your food intake. When you get to the G Factor Rules for success you'll find the details on how to do it.

Nutritional recommendations (minimum recommendations)
1. Multivitamin mineral
A good quality (not commercial bargain brands) multiple vitamin/mineral will be your basic support for appetite causes 1 and 2. This multi needs to contain:
  1. Chromium for blood sugar and appetite
  2. Vanadium for pancreatic support

3. B Complex for conversion of carbohydrates, enzyme production, stress control and blood sugar support.
4. Iodine, selenium, B6, magnesium and manganese for thyroid gland support.
5. Alpha lipoic acid for blood sugar support

2. Fiber product with eight ounces of water, 20 minutes before food optimum. Can be Glucomannan or Pectin fiber.

3. Essential fatty acids for appetite suppression optimally taken before each meal. In some people it can take 45 minutes or more for the EFA's to activate the production of CCK, but in many it can be much faster, even fewer than 5 minutes. Find out your perfect time through experimentation. At least 1200 mg will be necessary before each meal to produce sufficient CCK.

Stimulants
There is a great deal of controversy around the use of stimulants to control appetite. What dieter hasn't at least tried them? There are numerous types on the market. If you are tired and you have a slow metabolic rate, using a stimulant can make you feel more energetic and hopefully make you want to be more active. Some stimulants can burn very small amounts of fat without activity, but I still recommend increasing activity.

The most common stimulants today are caffeine and Guaranine. Guaranine is so similar to caffeine that only a sophisticated lab test can tell them apart. Guaranine comes from a plant called Guarana, which is unique to Brazil. The natives there chew the leaves for quick energy. Although both stimulants are naturally occurring, not everyone does well with these. If you are sensitive to stimulants, then avoid them, plain and simple. If you have high blood pressure or poor cardiovascular health, don't use stimulants.

Some people will benefit from their use but some people will release a stress hormone called cortisol, and those people may store fat as a result of that release. Those people should avoid caffeine in all forms; coffee, tea, soft drinks, and chocolate.

Theobromine and theophylline are among the least-known stimulants. Theophylline and its close relatives aminophylline, caffeine and chocolate, are members of the methylxanthine group of chemicals. Caffeine was the first of this group to be found helpful to asthmatic humans but had some unpleasant side effects. Other derivatives were quickly produced in hope of minimizing side effects and maximizing the airway relaxant properties that are so helpful in airway disease. Theophylline works well as a bronchial aid and has been made into a prescription drug. Natural theophylline available in dietary supplements is far less powerful.

Theobromine, along with an herb called rhodiola rosea, can also have a positive effect on your mood and sense of well-being. Most people agree that happiness is a good thing.

There are many other dietary ingredients that can stimulate metabolic function, but that would take up too much space to discuss them all here.

Those who can benefit from stimuli still should not rely on them. Chronic use can cause metabolic weight set point in some (not all) to adjust downward and, therefore, make it harder to maintain weight, let alone lose weight. It is always prudent, unless of course you have medical reasons not to exercise, to increase your activity levels everyday and stay active all your life. The chapter on exercise in this book will give you some easy, zero cost ways to exercise no matter where you are.

Psychological stimuli (the fourth cause)
In some cases the psychological stimuli, such as depression, causes the brain to need certain chemicals to be produced to fight that feeling. Some foods such as chocolate contain nutrients that contribute to the production of serotonin and, therefore, assist in many cases of depression. The problem is the amount of these nutrients per pound is simply too low to make a difference for most depression sufferers. This is why some people will binge on chocolate and still not get enough.

This is one of the many cases that a dietary supplement would make sense. Of course, the easy thing to do is take a drug, and too many doctors are fond of prescribing anti-depressants; but if your depression is linked to hormones, such as an imbalance or insufficiency of the female reproductive system, the right dietary supplements are very often the best and safest decision. Your body makes hormones from foods you eat, not from drugs. Plant hormones, known as phytohormones (from the Greek word phuton) have to combine with particular vitamins, minerals and essential fatty acids to become hormones in you.

The healthiest populations in terms of breast and prostate cancers on average consume more phytoestrogen than other populations. They eat between 20 and 80 mgs daily whereas Americans consume between 1-3 mgs daily on average.[27]

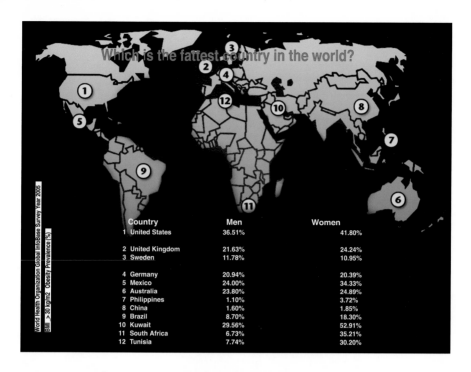

Country	Men	Women
1 United States	36.51%	41.80%
2 United Kingdom	21.63%	24.24%
3 Sweden	11.78%	10.95%
4 Germany	20.94%	20.39%
5 Mexico	24.00%	34.33%
6 Australia	23.80%	24.89%
7 Philippines	1.10%	3.72%
8 China	1.60%	1.85%
9 Brazil	8.70%	18.30%
10 Kuwait	29.56%	52.91%
11 South Africa	6.73%	35.21%
12 Tunisia	7.74%	30.20%

World Health Organization Global InfoBase Survey Year 2005
BMI > 30 kg/m2   Obesity Prevalence (%)

Glycemic Chart

Low	Medium	High
Skim milk	Banana	Watermelon
Plain Yogurt	Pineapple	Dried dates
Soy beverage	Raisins	Instant mashed potato
Apple/plum/oranges	New potatoes	Parsnips
Sweet potato	Popcorn	Rutabaga
Oat bran bread	Split pea or green pea soup	White rice
All-Bran™	Brown rice	Honey
Converted or Parboiled rice	Couscous	Rice Krispies™
Pumpernickel bread	Basmati rice	Cheerios
Al dente (firm) pasta	Shredded wheat cereal	Bagel, white
Lentils/kidney/baked beans	Whole wheat bread	Soda crackers
Chick peas	Stone ground rye bread	Jellybeans
Cashews	Table Sugar (sucrose)	French fries
Nuts	Sweet corn	Cookies
Ice cream (one scoop)	Cooked carrots	Processed juice
Meat, fowl, fish		Beer

1988

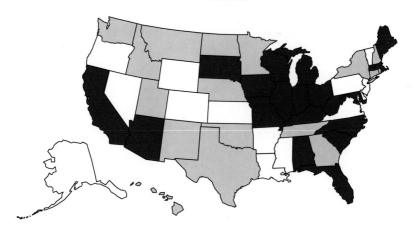

Obesity Trends Among U.S. Adults
1992

1996

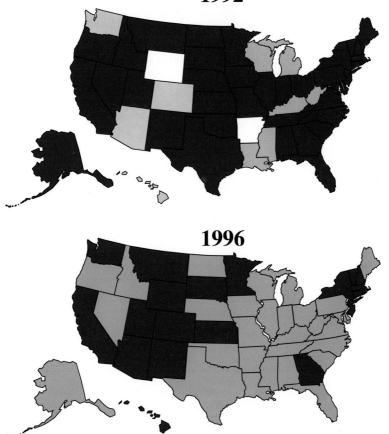

2000

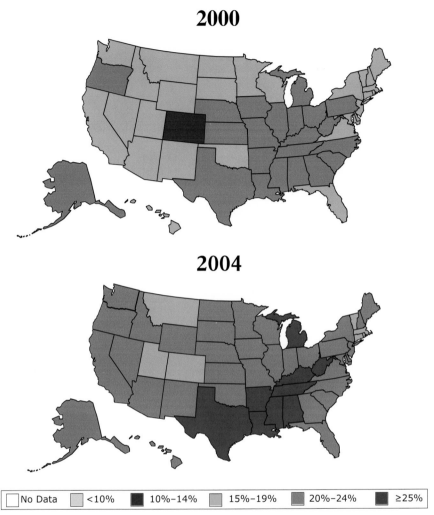

2004

| No Data | <10% | 10%–14% | 15%–19% | 20%–24% | ≥25% |

BMI ≥30, or about 30 lbs overweight for 5'4" person

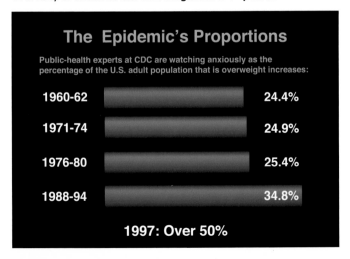

The Epidemic's Proportions

Public-health experts at CDC are watching anxiously as the percentage of the U.S. adult population that is overweight increases:

1960-62	**24.4%**
1971-74	**24.9%**
1976-80	**25.4%**
1988-94	**34.8%**

1997: Over 50%

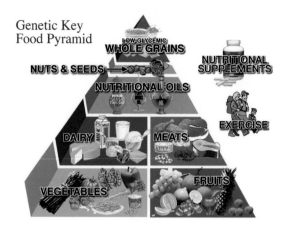

New USDA Low fat Pyramid

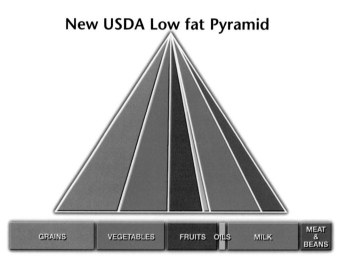

Original USDA Low fat Pyramid

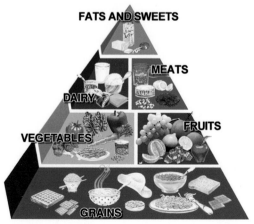

Additional scientific evidence, from cellular biology experiments, animal studies, and limited human Ingram clinical studies are consistent with the epidemiologic findings [28,29,30] Since the human body was designed to eat food, not drugs; and since the body was designed to produce all hormones as needed from particular foods, it makes sense to alter your diet and use dietary supplements, rather than drugs wherever possible.

The fourth, and less significant reason, is psychological stimuli. In most cases that has to be dealt with in a highly personal way.

Sleep (the fifth cause) and appetite control

If you deprive yourself of sleep, problems will occur. First, is the obvious, you are tired. If you are tired during the day, your brain will make you hungry for high glycemic foods, so that you can get quick surges in energy. You will stay tired until either you get some good sleep, or your adrenal glands kick in and you get your so-called second wind. The stressing of your adrenals is not good. You will keep snacking on high glycemic foods until the adrenals kick in, and then you won't be able to get to sleep and it starts all over again.

Also you replenish vital chemistry in your brain while you sleep and you need those chemicals to fight depression, as well as have clarity of thought and good memory function. So, get some sleep!

Chapter 7
Why do you hit plateaus and how to overcome them?

The Thrifty Gene, Obesity & Diabetes

In 1962, under the title ``Diabetes Mellitus: A 'thrifty' genotype rendered detrimental by `progress'," Dr. James Neel proposed the idea that the basic defect in diabetes mellitus was a quick insulin trigger. He suggested that this trigger was an asset to our tribal hunter-gatherer ancestors with their intermittent, sometimes feast-or-famine alimentation, since it should have minimized renal loss of precious glucose.[46]

In general, it is believed that the Thrifty Gene is most commonly found in what are considered to be older races. This gene is common in a higher percentage of Afro-Africans than any other race, but is found, to some degree, in all races. Interestingly, Neel seemed to be on to something because tests do indeed show that this gene plays a role in obesity and diabetes.[12,46]

Populations that carry this gene and who eat their traditional diets (low glycemic) have incredibly low incidence of heart disease, diabetes and obesity. When these same populations add "modern food" they become victims of all three diseases in disproportionately high numbers.[12,46]

If you possess the Thrifty Gene you are going to need to eat Low G or pay the price in health, fat gain, and a shorter life span. Your probability of becoming a diabetic, with all its associated problems, developing heart disease, hypertension or stroke, is, significantly high if you eat high G foods. It's not just about looking good and losing fat; its about your life!

Low fat but high G foods are poison to someone who has the Thrifty Gene.

The USDA Low fat food pyramid is based more on economics than anything else. Grain as a staple is a very recent addition to the human diet and is not natural to humans. Humans were initially hunter-gathers, without farming and food refinement technologies, and had no breads, pastas or refined high glycemic foods. The new low glycemic food pyramid makes sense for everyone, and it is far more natural to the human system.

Please take a look (at the center of the book) at my Genetic Key food pyramid and compare it to the original USDA food pyramid used for many years, while Americans began to really put on the fat. Its creation and use coincided with low fat and low cholesterol theories, but did not take into account the glycemic index. Obesity has gotten worse since its introduction and shows no sign of improvement.

Now look at their newest USDA pyramid. The USDA has changed their pyramid but it is still based on low fat. It still recommends that the majority of the daily diet should be high G grains and cereals, and look at how much milk it recommends. This pyramid is still wrong, still unhealthful, and will contribute to heart disease, diabetes and obesity. Moreover, the new pyramid looks like an advertisement for both corporate grain farming conglomerates and the American Milk Producers Association. Whose side is the USDA on anyway? It is still based on outdated information. Low fat foods are useless and even dangerous if they are high G!

The metabolic weight set point
This is not a discussion of plateaus while dieting. Those will happen and there are ways to overcome them. This is about genes. There is a theory accepted by many (including me), but not rigorously tested, that says all of us have a point at which our bodies want to settle weight-wise. At a given age and, of course, based on our genetics there will be a weight that our bodies do not want to go below, no matter what we try, short of dangerous methods such as starvation or surgery. Most diligent dieters have hit that point at some time and were frustrated because they wanted to weigh fewer pounds or kilos and weren't thinking about healthy body composition.

The theory follows the Thrifty gene theory to some extent. It goes on to say that it is an ancient survival mechanism to keep our hunter-gather ancestors from starving in between finding food in their wanderings. If the theory is correct (and I believe it is) then severe calorie restriction would make the weight set point intractable.

I have seen patients who were diligent and not cheating, who had over come plateaus in their diets but reached a point at which nothing was going to budge them one ounce lighter. Muscle mass and bone mass have weight. Even if you get yourself down to the percent body fat of a top athlete, you may not be able to get lighter without breaking down vital healthy tissue, including bone and muscle. Remember, it's not about how much you weigh, it's about how lean you are, and your percent of body fat.

So the best thing you can do is stay away from that darn scale! Use the measurement recommendations in this book. As you get healthier with less fat, you will be slimmer but you may not weigh whatever you thought you should.

Muscle weighs approximately 3 times more than fat per inch. So you can be many sizes smaller, be much healthier, and weigh more than you expected. With this in mind, don't worry too much about that weight set point.

As you get healthier with less fat, you will be slimmer but you may not weigh whatever you thought you should. Muscle weighs approximately 3 times more than fat per inch.

The crucial role of antioxidants

When people think about losing body fat and getting lean they rarely think about nutritional support. One of the reasons people plateau, is that we store toxins in our fat cells. This book is not about toxins so I will be brief and recommend that you read another one of my books called *How To Survive on a Toxic Planet,* if you are interested in the full details. In that book I cover antioxidants extensively.

These toxins cause free radical oxidative stress. Oxidative stress on metal is called rust. You don't rust, but what happens to your cells when they are attacked by free radicals isn't pretty and it isn't healthy.

We are taking these free radical causing toxins into the body in miniscule amounts 24 hours a day in air, water, and food. Unfortunately, we begin to take them in literally when we are in our mother's womb. Scientists have found disease-causing toxins in the snow, air, ice, and water of the North Pole, and fatty tissues of penguins at the South Pole. Humans tested all over planet Earth have been found to have toxins in their blood. There is literally no place in the 21st century that is toxin free.[24]

Naturally occurring toxins have always existed, but before the age of synthetic chemistry, which started about 1930, there were almost no synthetic toxins on the planet. Since that time there are more than 75,000 synthetic chemicals registered with the U.S. Environmental Protection Agency (EPA) alone. Many of these are known to cause diseases as serious as cancers, and many thousands of others are suspected to cause disease, but full testing has not yet been completed.[24]

The majority of these toxins are undetectable to the human sensory system. Since we do not see, smell, or taste them; and since the intake of them is so subtle, we do not notice any symptoms associated with them. When we convert fat as energy (some say burn fat), we release more toxins than our bodies antioxidant capacity. The brain will make you stop burning fat until your antioxidants can catch up and get you back on an even playing field.[24]

Free radicals—as long as they are controlled by antioxidants—cause no damage to the body. That's because the human body was designed to cope with a normal amount of free radical release during energy production, using antioxidants that come from fruits and vegetables, as well as, chemicals made in the body, such as glutathione. We no longer live in the world we were designed to live in. These environmental stresses have created a situation where our body's normal mechanisms for creating glutathione and utilizing antioxidants from foods are inadequate to protect us from these stresses. This results in fatigue, lethargy, and lack of clarity of thought, illness, disease, and premature aging and even premature death.[24]

The more stress, the greater the demand for organic fuel just to maintain an even playing field. This is why I recommend the best antioxidant supplement you can get, not just vitamins A, C or E, but a full complex. I recommend this for every human being, but if you are dieting and you are a Type GK 4 or GK 5, expect to plateau often unless you have sufficient antioxidants each day. Toxins that cause disease and death in humans are stored in fat cells.[24] With this in mind, the more stored fat you have the greater the probability of having health challenges due to toxins and the greater the need for antioxidants when the plateaus are happening.

A note on intestinal bypass surgery
I have seen patients who had this surgery and, at first, had dramatic success but over time became obese again. Why? It's simple, they became obese by eating high G foods. Either they didn't want to give them up, or they had been advised to eat low fat but high G foods. The mechanism will still go awry even if you have had a bypass. High G foods cause you to rise out of the GK zone and that results in stored body fat in type, GK 4 or GK 5 people - the people who have trouble with their weight. Surgery has its dangers and altering the way your body digests foods is a very bad idea, so don't even think about it.

The Genetic Key Diet

The

GENETIC KEY

Diet

The Key to Unlock a Lean Body & a Long Healthy Life

by Dr. Steve Nugent

Chapter 8
The History of Glycemic indexing and the Glycemic load

Before I explain the concept of the glycemic index and the glycemic load further, I want to give you the history that led up to it.

Oh Canada!
The few people who are familiar with glycemic indexing probably don't know how that concept really started. In 1979, a Canadian researcher named Jean Renaud was doing research on diabetes and obesity. He found that hyperinsulinism (very high insulin responses) was present in all cases of obesity regardless of body type. This triggered some important research by many scientists.[1]

In 1981 Dr. David Jenkins, a professor of nutrition at the University of Toronto, Canada, developed the concept of the glycemic index. He was also doing this to help diabetics. Whether he was influenced by Renaud's findings, I do not know for sure, but Jenkins is the man who created the GI as we know it. His study, titled "Glycemic Index of Foods: A Physiological Basis for Carbohydrate Exchange," started the proverbial snowball rolling downhill. I feel every book written since then, that refers to the GI in anyway, owes something to Jenkins.[2]

Since then many hundreds of studies have been done in the United Kingdom, France, Italy, Canada, and Australia that have shown more than sufficient evidence to prove the value of the glycemic index. The U.S. is simply not with the program yet. Harvard and The American Journal of Clinical Nutrition have published several important papers that appear to go unnoticed by the U.S., government, medical authorities and the media. The Harvard studies are very convincing, yet the U.S. still remains in the "Dark Ages" as far as diet for diabetes, heart disease, and fat loss is concerned.

In 1987, a Frenchman named Michel Montignac, having no medical or scientific background, devised a method called the Montignac method. His method is a variation on the glycemic theme, geared first for fat loss and then diabetes and heart disease. His concept wasn't introduced in the U.S. until 1999. He wrote a book called Eat Yourself Slim that has sold 15 million copies around the world, mostly in Europe, with very little impact unfortunately, in the U.S. France did adapt glycemic indexing and their statistics for heart disease are the best of any modern nation. Could their diet be a factor?

In 1996, a now famous Canadian cardiologist named Jean Dumesnil, who after losing 46 pounds himself on the Montignac method, decided to find out why it worked. His limited study was done at the Quebec Heart Institute at Laval University in Quebec City, Canada.

The Laval's researchers recruited 12 obese men from the general public. They averaged a Body Mass Index of 33. For three weeks, they came to the hospital for their meals. They were put on three different programs: the American Heart Association diet (low fat); the Montignac Method, and the third was a combination of the two. At no time were they told which diet or even the kind of diet they were on.

The men in the study who succeeded were using Montignac's version of glycemic indexing and they reported feeling very satisfied with the amount of food they ate. These men later learned that they had eaten 25 percent fewer calories than on the other two diets, yet none of the diets restricted the quantities of food at all. The test subjects ate less because employing low GI correctly reduces appetite as well as insulin responses.

According to Dr. Dumesnil, using this form of dieting had a favorable effect on cholesterol and insulin levels, as well as, fat loss. Although he wasn't exactly sure what the mechanism of action was at the time he reported. Dr. Jenkins, the inventor of the Glycemic Index, is not in full agreement with the Montignac Method.

In 1997, Dr. Jorge Salmeron and Dr. Walter Willett at the Harvard School of Public Health conducted the famous Nurses' Health Study of 121,700 U.S. female registered nurses over many years. It showed that women who ate a low glycemic, high-fiber diet had two-and-half times less risk of developing diabetes. This was published in JAMA, yet most medical doctors in America still recommend low fat.[3]

Harvard University publishes several newsletters on health related topics. The December 2000 issue of the *Harvard Women's Health Watch* (*HWHW*) recommended that consumers should place fresh fruits and non-starchy vegetables at the base of their Food Guide Pyramid, along with whole grains and beans. These foods are rich in nutrients and contain fiber, which slows digestion and moderates blood glucose levels. This is the low glycemic principal.[8]

In the 2001 issue of the *Harvard Women's Health Watch* (*HWHW*) there was an article titled "Glycemic Load, Diet, and Health". The article did a good job summarizing the concept of glycemic load or GL. I highly recommend their online newsletters although there was an error in this one. They failed to factor fiber into their calculation. Typing errors occur even in the best of publications written by the finest minds. I still recommend it for an explanation of the GL.[7] Because of its obvious benefits in controlling blood glucose, the glycemic load is now the focus of dietary recommendations for diabetics in the U.K., Australia, Canada, and France. While the U.S. has not yet adopted such recommendations, Harvard experts were hoping, as far back as the year 2000, that we would see "Low Glycemic Load" on product labels, just as we now see packages that read "Low Cholesterol". However, at this time, only Australia has begun labeling foods as low, moderate, or high glycemic, thanks largely to the efforts of Professor Brand-Miller and her team.

Professor Jennie Brand-Miller was the lead author of a book in 1996 on diabetes, heart disease and weight reduction.[47] The North American edition of that book was released in 1999. I was very hopeful then that the U.S. would catch on, but it didn't happen. That particular book has sold more than 1.7 million copies around the world since 1996, but it had very little impact in the U.S. The book is written in nine languages. If you consider the total population of the U.S. alone, over 294 million, (as of July 2005) then total the populations of all those other countries, clearly it has had almost no impact in the big picture of fat loss, heart disease, or diabetes. Only a tiny fraction of the world's population is aware of this information, for most people (especially Americans) it is totally new! Her work continues and her team at the University of Sydney continues to lead in this area, although Harvard is moving fast and furious in this direction.

I cannot applaud Professor Brand-Miller enough for her work, and I am so pleased to say that the Australian government is open to any science that will reduce health issues in their nation. For this reason, Professor Brand-Miller has made her greatest impact in Australia. The GI symbol program initiated by her work was launched in Australia in 2002 to help consumers identify the GI of foods. Consumers can be certain; foods that carry the symbol are guaranteed to have been properly tested by an accredited laboratory. We definitely need that in every country.

Even though Harvard is pushing for it here in the U.S., the U.S. health and medical officials seem uninterested, even resistant in many cases. Perhaps if health care in the U.S. wasn't privatized the government might have a greater interest. In Australia, they realize rising health care costs are going to bankrupt their socialized medicine system, and heart disease and diabetes are very expensive to treat. The studies are clear-low G eating reduces diabetes, heart disease, and is the most efficient way to shed body fat.

Dr. Walter Willett originated the glycemic load and introduced that concept to the public in 2001. GL is a more accurate measure of insulin response to foods than GI.[4]

In 1998, when I created my first material for the GI system, I used a traffic signal idea- green for go (low G), yellow for caution (moderate G), and red for stop, (high G). Many are doing that now on websites and printed material. It would be great to have all food labels color-coded that way for public health in all countries.

It wasn't until March 2005 that the USA Today Newspaper finally said that GI is in and low carb is out. Even so, most everyone still isn't on the program yet. In fact, in February 2006, there was another article that represented incomplete data but was written to say that low GI foods didn't change blood sugar etc. Complete and comprehensive examination of the data does prove that low G does exactly what its proponents say it does.

As I have stated, there have been hundreds of scientific papers since Jenkins invented the index. Yet, the public is almost totally unaware of it and health officials in the U.S. keep pushing low fat and low cal. Science moves slowly, my friends, but when a change effects someone's ego, status, or bank account it can be even worse.

Ok, now that you have the basic history, we can move on.

Chapter 9
How do I use the Genetic Key to get into the GK Zone?

Benefits of a Low G diet, according to the University of Sydney, New South Wales, Australia, and Harvard University experts
* Low GI diets help people lose and control weight
* Low GI diets increase the body's sensitivity to insulin
* Low GI carbs improve diabetes control
* Low GI carbs reduce the risk of heart disease
* Low GI carbs reduce blood cholesterol levels
* Low GI carbs reduce hunger and keep you fuller for longer
* Low GI carbs prolong physical endurance

We have discussed the history and the reasons why other diets fail. We have talked about metabolic types and now it's time to talk about what you're going to eat, to get into, and stay in the GK Zone.

Forget what you have heard or what you have learned about low fat, low cal and low carb. Forget the "all soup", all "ice cream" or all "peach diet". Forget the gimmicks. It's time to learn about the last diet you'll ever need. Getting into the GK Zone.

The rules are so simple that anyone can understand and use them faithfully. The question is, when you understand them, will you choose wisely? Will you choose to follow these rules for life? Or will you choose to be fat and unhealthy? Ultimately the choice is yours alone.

Understanding The Genetic Key
In our high-tech society, science is always looking for ways to improve upon nature. Sometimes this can be done, but when it comes to diet, science has repeatedly failed. Why? The human body is a highly complex organism that was designed to eat foods that occur in nature. Tampering with nature's delicate balance usually results in negative consequences. The more we refine our foods or encourage diets that do not have a balance of naturally occurring nutrients and fibers, the worse our health becomes as a society. Balance is the key to wellness and the information you are about to read reflects this.

The Genetic Key is more than a diet. It is an opportunity for anyone to learn how to obtain and maintain healthy body composition and, therefore, lay the foundation for achieving optimal health.

What is Glycemic indexing?
As defined earlier, the Genetic Key Diet principles encompass glycemic indexing, the glycemic load, and the glucagon mechanism factored in with our genetic type. The glycemic index and glycemic load aren't new. I didn't invent them, although I did create the world's first system including supplements and exercise based on its principals back in 1998 and launched to the world in 1999. The newest science is showing that low G (low glycemic) diets reduce the risk of heart disease and diabetes. Too bad U.S. authorities have not yet embraced the healthiest diet for the world.

Many books have been published on the subject and the authors, although in general agreement, differ in many areas. It is not my intention to reinvent the wheel, but rather to offer the Genetic Key Diet as one component of what I feel is the most intelligent approach to a total lifestyle change for improved health in virtually every area, not just fat loss.

The glycemic index is about measuring how much a given food raises your blood sugar. This is important because the rate at which your blood sugar rises after eating is extremely important and, until recently, an ignored factor in the total equation of weight management.

When you consume a high G food, it causes your blood sugar to rise above normal and this, in turn, causes your insulin to rise. This increase of blood sugar has many negative affects above the obvious. Foods that raise blood sugar abnormally increase your appetite, contribute to mood swings, diabetes, and heart disease, as well as, increase stored fat by increasing triglyceride production.

Some have asked me why the glycemic index numbers vary from book to book and study to study. I hope that eventually the authorities at the World Health Organization will come to recognize this as a new standard for health, but in the meantime, there are variances in methods of testing. The variance is slight in most cases, however. You may, as an example, have one reference list a peach as 26 or 30 or white potatoes as 85 or 100. Don't waste time splitting hairs. The peach in that example would still be low G and the potato would still be high G.

The measurements are somewhat complex but basically it works like this. A test group is assembled; they draw blood to test for sugar before eating a particular food and then again 2 hours and in some studies 4 and 6 hours after eating the food. Each person on earth is biochemically and genetically unique so each may have a slightly different number. The group then is averaged in most cases and that is published as the index of a given food.

So, currently expect that there will be differences, but let's go back to our previous paragraph. The glycemic index is not cumulative. A rise in blood sugar is cumulative to a certain level, but a rise in insulin is continuously cumulative. Sound confusing? This is why we must have a diet based on all factors that is geared toward nature's diet and is balanced. Once again, this is why I made my G Factor Rules, don't bog yourself down with details. I am supplying details only to provide information for better understanding. I want you to feel comfortable with the system, but please just follow the G Factor Rules and keep it simple.

On the Glycemic Index (GI) foods are listed as high, moderate, or low. There is some disagreement among authors and researchers as to which level represents high, moderate, or low. For the purpose of this guide, we will use the following guidelines.

0-54 is low G
55-70 is moderate G
71 and above is high G

Some authors show white potatoes as low as 85 and some at 100, this is due primarily to slight variations in testing methods. Whether white potatoes are 85 or 100 is not important. What is important is that they are high glycemic any way you look at it, and they need to be avoided with rare exceptions, which I will cover. Don't get tangled up in all the details and viewpoints. You should also note that this index is based on glucose not white bread.

The G Factor Rules for Success
1 Eat foods in their natural state wherever possible.
2 Eat foods that are comparatively difficult to digest.
3 Eat foods that are high in fiber.
4 Time your food intake.
5 Avoid white foods*.
6 Don't use artificial sweeteners.
7 Drink sufficient water*

7 Rules for Success (explained)

1. Eat foods in their natural state wherever possible (obviously this does not include meats and foods, which would be dangerous to eat raw). I am referring to foods like carrots, for example. What is the natural state of a carrot? Raw, of course. When they are eaten raw it is safe, natural, and the way we were designed to eat them. When they are raw they also fit my second rule and that is raw foods are harder to digest. They also fit my third rule that is eat foods that are higher in fiber. Raw carrots are low G, but cooked carrots (not their natural state) are moderate G.

2. Eat foods that are comparatively difficult to digest. (The harder it is to digest typically the lower glycemic it is). I didn't say impossible, nor did I say make yourself uncomfortable. The principle is simple, the harder it is to digest, the longer it takes to convert to blood sugar. This minimizes insulin reactions and you can then maximize your conversion of food to energy over time for sustained energy and minimize the amount that converts to fat. Cooked carrots are very easy to digest so their index is much higher than raw.

3. Eat foods that are high in fiber. Fiber ranges from hard to digest to impossible to digest. Impossible is actually good for humans. It not only helps with a feeling of fullness it also helps to clean our colons and that is crucial to good health. The higher the fiber, the more absorbent of fats, and the slower your digestion, so the lower the glycemic index is. A good example would be breads. Highly refined white bread has had the fiber so broken down that it is virtually useless for colon health. It is soft, mushy, and easy to digest. It is not in its natural state (rule number 1) and it is white (rule number 5). Whole grain bread with seeds is as close as bread can get to the natural state of grain. Depending on the grain and the seeds it could be low or moderate G, but not high. So, yes, you can have bread but not highly refined, high G bread. Unlike what appears in the USDA Food Pyramid, the base of the pyramid should be made of low G vegetables and some fruits, not high G breads and cereals. In fact, it is the high glycemic base of the pyramid that has probably contributed to more excess body fat, heart disease, and diabetes than any other single factor.

4. Time your food intake. It is very important to your overall health, but particularly important to achieving a lean body to keep your blood sugar balanced. Skipping meals may save calories, but that will eventually backfire on you as your body will perceive a state of starvation and reduce the rate at which you convert your stored fats to insure that you will not starve. Genetic scientists now refer to the "Thrifty Gene" as the culprit. Snacking is good if it's with the right foods. It helps to keep your blood sugar balanced and this helps to control appetite, as well as maximize your ability to convert stored fat as energy. Your snacks need to fit a certain set of guidelines, however. It would be ideal if we could get everyone to snack on fresh fruit or vegetables that are low glycemic, such as peaches or celery, but this isn't always convenient, so under snacks I will give you some suggestions. For now, as an example, a half dozen almonds eaten every 2 hours between meals should help the average person maintain a reasonable level of blood sugar. Once again, this varies with each individual to some extent. Don't go too long between meals. It is true that several small meals properly balanced and indexed are far healthier than three heavy meals. Remember our discussion of the human design and our ancestral diet? We'll discuss this further under meal plans.

5. Avoid white foods. There are exceptions to every rule. If you look hard, enough white foods tend to be high glycemic. Raw cauliflower is an exception; white potatoes are the highest (85-100) on the glycemic index. White potatoes are a starchy complex, and those starches convert to glucose rapidly. Additionally, they are very easy to digest (that violates rule number 2) and contain very little fiber (that violates rule number 3). All grain products from bread to pastas (if white) are to be avoided because most of them are high and few rare ones are moderate. Egg white and cauliflower are obviously low G, so use common sense when I talk about avoiding white food, it means breads and cereals.

6. Don't use artificial sweeteners. There is preliminary evidence that artificial sweeteners may slow the fat burning process by confusing the normal chemical signals to the brain that are normally associated with sweet tastes. Sweet tastes also increase your appetite of sweets. There is no evidence that they really assist in fat loss, and there is also an increasing body of evidence that some artificial sweeteners may have harmful effects on the body. Since the evidence is still in question on artificial sweeteners, I recommend they not be used. You may think now that you can't live without sweeteners, but you'd be surprised how little you desire those dangerous substances once your body cleanses and balances. Suggestions and substitutions will be covered later.

7. Increase water intake. Water is the essence of life itself. Most people complain about drinking it but you simply cannot maintain proper balance without it. Water is vital for cleansing your body, maintaining proper hormonal balance, which is of course extremely important in weight management, and is vitally important in fat transport. The body of a male adult consists of approximately 60% water, while an adult female is approximately 50% water. This difference is because women in general have more fat tissue and less muscle than men do. The fat tissue typically contains only 20% water, while the muscles contains about 75% water. The content of water in other tissues also varies, from respectively 3% and 25% in the teeth-enamel and the bone-tissue, to 99% in the vitreous humor in the eye. Brain tissue is approximately 80% water, and blood is about 79% water. The body of an infant contains more water than the body of an adult, about 80%. Do not expect long-term success on any program without proper hydration. Drink filtered water and drink it constantly all day long.

At the center of the book you will find a chart of some foods that have been tested for their GI. The chart is color-coded like a traffic signal. As I present this information in cities around the world, I nearly always get the same questions from the audience. So I will answer those here. By answering these, it helps to reinforce the concept of metabolic types and the ten rules. I explain the GI and the GL only for those who need it. The G Factor Rules are really the practical guide for everyday food choices.

FAQ's regarding GI Food Chart

Let's talk about the foods listed, on the GI Food Chart found at the center of the book to help you further understand the concept. Remember what I said earlier that many people with weight problems are looking for ways to keep eating the foods that made them fat. I am very sorry to report that foods that are bad for your metabolic type must be avoided. There are no miracles to allow you to abuse yourself and still be healthy and lean, if you are a G4 or G5.

Let's go over some of the foods in the chart that may, at first glance, puzzle some of you. Some who read and understand the G Factor Rules will know instantly why these foods are rated the way they are.

The sample foods listed are based on 100 gram or 3.5 ounce serving sizes. The reason is some foods, when you increase the serving size, you increase the glycemic load beyond the point at which it is still low G. Don't get stressed; I will explain the load in a minute.

Remember my examples of white potatoes and sweet potatoes. It's all about fiber. So white is high G and sweet is low G. That means, if you have two sweet potatoes, you will create a load. But you need only one right?

If you don't like a food that has been listed, pork for example or you have philosophical or religious reasons for avoiding a particular food then look at the foods you do like and substitute. Common sense will have to be employed sometimes. The overwhelming majority of people will choose foods from all groups without restriction and I want this to work for everyone.

Honey
Q: Why is honey listed as high? Isn't honey a healthy sugar substitute?
A: Honey is good for you in small amounts, but the primary sugar in honey is sucrose. Yes, the same molecule as table sugar and honey is liquid so it is slightly easier to digest than granulated sucrose. Remember G Factor Rule number 2? Honey has other benefits, but it is not a better sugar or sugar substitute.

Rice

Q : How can white rice be high glycemic? Why are there skinny Orientals, don't they eat white rice?

A: I discussed biochemical individuality and adaptation to food earlier. If you are Oriental you likely can eat white rice without deleterious effects; but if you're German you can't. Why? Orientals have adapted to that food over the centuries, but it is a very new food for other cultures and they have not adapted yet.

If your genetic group <u>has not</u> had many centuries to adapt to a food, your body will probably not process it correctly and you'll pay a price when you eat it.

All of us had hunter-gatherer ancestors. We know that today's hunter-gatherer groups get 1% or less of their diets in wild grains. Scientists suspect it was always that way before farming. Today, wild brown rice is low G for everyone regardless of genetics or metabolic type.

Potatoes

Q: Why are mashed white potatoes slightly lower than baked white potatoes?

A: Simple, these mashed potatoes had some milk added to them and milk contains both fat and protein, which are both 0 G, so that lowers the total index very slightly. The bottom line, however, is that they are both still high G, regardless. White potatoes are not native to any continent, except America. The English Jamestown colonists brought them back to England as gifts from the Indians along with tobacco. Some gift. The Spanish conquistadors brought some back to Spain as well. Nobody in mainland Europe wanted to eat the ugly things that grew underground, and for the Spanish these might be evil foods too, because they were favorites of the pagan Indians. The English decided to have them grown in Ireland to feed the Irish because they were hardy plants, and it didn't matter to the English court what the Irish ate. Over time the Irish became totally dependent on the potato but not long enough to become genetically adapted to them. It is almost impossible to find any descendants of the Native Americans who were adapted to the potato, so, for all practical purposes consider them high G for everyone.

Yes, I love them too. Everyone I know does. Since I changed my lifestyle to Low G in 1998, I have not eaten one. I miss the aroma, taste, and texture -- I love them; but life is full of choices and I choose to live healthy. So I keep low G. You cannot make excuses for unhealthy foods. Ultimately, the choice is yours, I hope you choose wisely.

Psychology can help or hinder. If a food makes you fat no matter how good it tastes it is BAD! Stop saying things like, "Oh but white potatoes are soooooo good." Using a positive phrase to reinforce a negative food is counterproductive to your health. So stop saying a food is good if you know it makes you fat or contributes to ill health.

Watermelon
Q: Why is watermelon high?
A: It is water, sugar, and almost no fiber to slow the conversion of the sugar, so it fails G Factor Rule 2 and 3.

Processed or fresh squeezed juice
Q: Why is processed juice moderate and natural juice low?
A: Simple, G Factor Rules 1, 2 and 3. G Factor Rule 1 Eat foods in their natural state wherever possible. G Factor Rule 2: Eat foods that are comparatively difficult to digest, and G Factor Rule 3: Eat foods that are higher in fiber. Fresh squeezed has natural pulp and that's fiber, which as you know is very difficult, if not impossible, to digest. Processed nearly always has sugar added to sweeten the taste. The sweetest oranges are typically sold for eating as a whole fruit. Stick with the rules, my friends.

White foods and grains
Also note the theme of white foods being high G. Remember what I said about thinking in absolutes? It is not that you can't have grain products, but you must select those that are Low G if you are a G5 and low or moderate G if you are a metabolic type G4. The other metabolic types should still avoid high G foods, as they are bad for your health.

If you need to get started fast on your diet and burn the fat inches off without delay, then avoid all moderate G foods until you have lost the first few pounds, but remember that balance is the key to wellness. It is important that you consume some carbohydrates daily; 0 carb dieting is unhealthy and will trigger your survival mechanisms, resulting in slowing your metabolic rate and making long-term weight management more difficult.

The rules work, and if you use them with common sense, you don't need to have the numbers for every food in the world. Hopefully this section has helped you to understand them better.

Here is another example to help you understand how simple this is, and that you don't need to do math or know the index of every possible food. I have mentioned nuts often. Some will say, "Yes, but what's the index of this nut or that nut?" Fifty grams of salted mixed nuts (you name them) has a GI of 24 (very Low G) and a GL of 4 (very Low G). Those 50 grams contain 17.3 grams of carbohydrates (this is not a low carb diet).

That's about 1.25 ounces of nuts and that is far more than I recommend for snacks. A typical can of nuts purchased at a grocery store is 6 ounces total. I recommend you snack on 6 nuts every two hours (or one hour) if you are hypoglycemic. Some may not need the extra blood sugar support, so if you don't need it, don't snack.

Also, the taste of salt and sugar both increase appetite. So salted and honey roasted nuts will simply make you want to keep eating. Follow G factor Rule 1: Eat foods in their natural state whenever possible.

Q: Nuts have fat -- especially cashews -- Can I eat cashews?
A: Yes, but not by the pound. Let's take a look at cashews. Because nuts of all types are hard to digest (G Factor Rule number 2) they are low GI and low GL and, therefore, Low G. Splitting hairs about roasted verses raw is irrelevant in terms of the G Factor, but they can effect appetite. So, yes, you can eat cashews, this is not a low fat diet. However, remember why I recommend nuts of any kind; it is in conjunction with appetite and blood sugar control, and you apply it as I have directed - 6 nuts, not 1.5 ounces or 6 ounces at a time. One cashew averages about 1.2 grams so 6 would be 7.2 grams and, as you can see from the chart below, both low GI and low GL and, therefore, Low G. Almonds are about one gram per piece.

This is important to G Factor Rule number 4: Time your food intake. Stop worrying about the math, my G Factor Rules work.

Food	Serving size	Glycemic index	Carbohydrates	Glycemic load
Cashews raw	50 grams	25	12.4	3
Cashews roasted and salted	50 grams	27	10.3	3
Cashews (organic) roasted and salted	50 grams	25	11.7	3

Almonds are what I recommend most because of the total net nutritional content. One ounce of almonds has 6 grams of protein, 3 grams of fiber, with only 1 gram of bad fat. Almonds help significantly to reduce appetite in concert with G Factor rules 2-4.

The Glycemic Load (Too much of a good thing?)
It is possible to have too much of a good thing. You can eat too much Low G
food and cause a glycemic load (**GL**). It's the load that measures the real stress
on your body, not the index alone. One GL unit is an indication of the effects of
1 gram of glucose on your insulin levels. It is, therefore, more accurate than the
GI alone and experts at Harvard, want to see it as our new standard. Relax, don't
panic, if you hate math or this seems confusing. Remember there are people who
not only want, but need, complex technical info. If you're not one of them, that's
ok, the 7 rules make choosing food dieting simple and easy and most people will
use them.

As you have learned in this book, the GI (glycemic index) is one aspect of the
G Factor, and it's a measure of how your blood sugar reacts to a given food. At
a certain volume of low G foods, you will create a load on pancreatic function
called the glycemic load. This is the measurement of true effect that any food
has on your insulin response. Mathematically you arrive at the GL by multiply-
ing the amount of carbohydrate contained in a specified serving size of the food
by the GI value of that food (with the use of glucose as the reference food),
which is then divided by 100. [44,3]

$$GL = \text{Carbohydrate grams x GI} \div 100$$

Low GL = 10 or less
Medium GL = 11- 19
High GL = 20 or more

Daily cumulative GL
Low GL < 80
High GL > 120

GL is typically summed up as the total of all the foods in a meal or an entire day
for study purposes. According to the University of Sydney at New South Wales,
Australia, under the leadership of Professor Jennie Brand-Miller, valuable
research on the GI and the GL tell us that a typical diet has about 100 GL units
per day and the average daily range is 60 – 180 GL. To be healthy, every metabolic type should stay below 120 daily GL, but if you're a G 5 you may have to
be around 60 to get rid of the stubborn fat.

University of Sydney has done fabulous work for human health, and their GI
database gives both GI & GL values of many foods, but a caution for those of

you who are not Australian. There are foods commercially available in many countries that have the same product name but different ingredients, which in some cases changes the G Factor.

Can unhealthy foods be low G?

Yes… The scientists at University of Sydney, just like the researchers at University of Toronto and Harvard are scientists first and foremost. When they test and report the GI or GL, they don't make value judgments; they simply report the facts. So you will see things on the lists that are low but not things I would necessarily recommend for your health.

One notable example would be artificial sweeteners or diet foods or drinks that contain artificial sweeteners. You already know my feelings on these. I believe they stimulate appetite and there is no evidence that they assist real fat loss. Moreover, they may be dangerous to your health, but at this time the jury is still out on that. These scientists make no comment about whether something is healthy, or unhealthy; simply high, moderate or low G. So if you feel a particular food or drink is bad for you, simply avoid it regardless of the index.

No math required

Most people don't like doing math and it isn't very convenient to stop and do a math equation before each food you eat. So I have included some quick reference examples of low, moderate, and high glycemic load foods. Notice how they correspond to the G Factor Rules. You don't need to complicate your life. Just use the G Factor Rules and common sense.

Note: The glycemic index is typically measured with very small amounts of a given food as in the chart in this book, whereas, the load factor is measured with greater amounts. That is how low G foods can become high G foods.

Glycemic load is clearly more accurate mathematically, however. I have counseled you in this book to eat slowly, time your food intake, and to eat smaller amounts more frequently while using fiber such as glucomanna or pectin to reduce appetite, leaving a feeling of fullness. To follow my system correctly, it is essential that you do this. Therefore, the glycemic load is of less importance than following the G Factor rules and my other guidelines.

Having said all that, I know there are some people who will still want to see some glycemic load examples, so they are listed below. Compare these to the list of low G foods color-coded in the center of the book and my 7 rules.

Low Glycemic Load
High-fiber fruits and vegetables (not including white potatoes)
Bran cereals (1 oz.)
Many legumes, including chickpeas, kidney beans, black beans, lentils, pinto beans
(5 oz. cooked, approx. 3/4 cup)

Medium Glycemic Load
Brown rice: 3/4 cup cooked
Oatmeal: 1 cup cooked
Bulgur wheat: 3/4 cup cooked
Rice cakes: 3 cakes
Whole grain breads: 1 slice
Whole-grain pasta: 1 1/4 cup cooked
No-sugar added fruit juices: 8 oz. (3.5 ounce was low G)

High Glycemic Load
Baked white potato
French fries
Refined cereal products: 1 oz.
Sugar-sweetened beverages: 12 oz.
Jelly beans: 10 large or 30 small
Candy bars: 1 2-oz. bar or 3 mini bars (some with high nut content are low)
Couscous: 1 cup cooked
Cranberry juice cocktail: 8 oz.
White basmati rice: 1 cup cooked
White-flour pasta: 1 1/4 cup cooked
Glycemic load categorization adapted from Foster-Powell K, Holt SH, Brand-Miller JC. International table of glycemic index and glycemic load values: 2002. Am J Clin Nutr. 2002; 76:5-56.

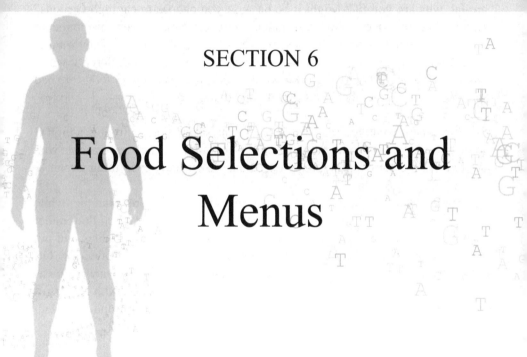

SECTION 6

Food Selections and Menus

The Key to Unlock a Lean Body & a Long Healthy Life

by Dr. Steve Nugent

Frequently Asked Questions on Food Selections

I have decided to answer the questions that always come up when people read my meal suggestions before you look at the menus. That will expedite your reading since you won't be pondering every unfamiliar entry.

Before we start, I want you to get focused and use some common sense. If you are fat, why are you fat? Might it be because you choose to eat high G foods? Hmm... Yes, that does sound reasonable. Yet every time I teach this course to doctors or laymen I always get those who aren't using their heads. They want to try to find a way to continue eating the wrong foods yet succeed. Sorry, it won't work and I wouldn't do it even if it would work, because high G foods are bad for your health, remember heart disease and diabetes?

So, think about what you really love. There is a strong possibility it is a high G food which have contributed to your current condition. As I observe people who are fighting the battle of the bulge, I see them do virtually everything wrong.

They select low fat but high G foods almost exclusively. For example, white bread or white dinner role, and cream soups made with white refined flour rather than cream. They select white potatoes rather than low G vegetables and put margarine on them rather than butter. They select a high G (but often low fat) salad dressing that has been sweetened artificially. They choose watermelon as their fruit. They have low fat, high G desserts and wash it down with a diet soft drink or lite beer. Why do they continue to fail? Once you understand the G factors -- it's obvious.

Lets look at the most frequently asked questions.

Question: Since fat is zero G, why have you recommended low fat foods to get me into the GK zone in some cases?
Answer: Fat, as mentioned earlier, is low G, but don't forget that fat grams are the most calorie-rich food, and keeping your daily fat low, not zero is a good idea.

Question: Can I use caffeinated beverages rather than water or vegetable juice?
Answer: Yes, but there are some things to know first. Caffeinated beverages are problematic for <u>some</u> dieters. They can cause the release of cortisol (an adrenal stress hormone). In some, this can cause fat to deposit on the waistline or hips. This is not the case for everyone, and for many people caffeine helps the con-

tinuous burn of fat by keeping up the metabolic rate. Only you know who you are in this regard. The majority of patients I observed over the years using caffeine or Guaranine received some mild short-term benefit to their metabolic rates that out-weighed the effects of any cortisol output. Generally speaking, however, the healthiest stimulant is exercise.

Question: Can I use diet sodas?
Answer: No! First, there is no evidence that diet sodas actually help you lose weight. That may surprise you, but it's true. Next, the jury is still out on the safety of sugar substitutes. In my opinion insufficient study has been done, even on aspartame, which was discovered way back in 1965. The anecdotal reports of side effects simply are too numerous to ignore. "Almost natural" isn't natural. I first wrote back in 1996 in my international newsletter (The Nugent Report) that I suspected that sugar substitutes (of all types) were causing weight gain because they increase your brains desire for sugar. Your brain and muscles must have sugar to function and if your sweet receptors detect a sweet taste but no actual sugar is going into your body, then your appetite for sweets increases.

Question: What should I do for a sweetener or sugar substitute?
Answer: I wouldn't use a sugar substitute. Sucrose (table sugar) is the most common sugar found in plants and required to run your body. Sucrose isn't bad, excess levels of it are bad. Your body requires the equivalent of ten teaspoons of sucrose in a normal day according to the USDA. That would include all you receive from all natural foods you eat, not adding spoons of sugar each day. Sucrose, surprisingly, is moderate on the index if you do not exceed 1 teaspoon during any 2-hour period. If you are any metabolic type other than G5, you can use it in moderation.

If you choose not to use sucrose, use Xylitol. Xylitol is low glycemic, natural and tastes great. It is a natural sugar, Xylose, that has been extracted from fruits or vegetables with an alcohol process. Anything that is extracted with an alcohol process ends in ol. Xylitol is as sweet as sucrose, has 33% fewer calories than sucrose, will not promote tooth decay, and won't raise your blood sugar. There are also studies that show it contributes to healthy teeth and bones, as well as reduces the incidence of ear infections in children.

Question: Can I use lime instead of lemon in my water?
Answer: Yes, but lemon is more efficient for cleansing the liver.

Question: Which nut or seed is the best choice for snacks?
Answer: Almonds are the best choice. All nuts and seeds, however, are low G.

Question: If I have trouble with dairy, can I use soymilk?
Answer: Yes, but read labels carefully. Many soymilks are artificially sweetened or have sugar added.

Question: If I have trouble with dairy, can I use tofu rather than cheese?
Answer: Yes.

Question: I noticed on the index that beer is very high glycemic. Is light beer different?
Answer: Sorry, it's not about calories, it is about the G Factors. Beer of any type, including the finest Old World Ale is still high G. Think about the G Factor Rules. It violates Rules 1, 2, and 3. There is reason for the phrase "beer belly".

Question: What alcohols can I drink?
Answer: Obviously, beer and ale are out, spirits have an index of 0 and a glycemic load of 0. Both red and white wine have an index of 0 and a glycemic load of 0. However, it is not a good idea to consume too much alcohol for a variety of reasons. The average person can do well with one glass of wine. The negative effects on liver and brain cells from over consumption of alcohol are well known. Red wine has some minor advantages over white wine or spirits. The antioxidant value of red wine is significant. The anti-platelet aggregation factor (APAF) is also noteworthy. APAF helps to keep sticky cells called platelets from clumping together which is good for circulation and heart health. When platelets clump they can block blood flow to the heart and brain. No solid data exists currently to explain why, but people who are chronically battling with their weight nearly always select beer or white wine. Lean people with healthy hearts tend, in general, to automatically select red wine, before they are educated on the benefits of it.

Question: What about other desserts?
Answer: Nature's desert is called fruit! What a concept. Most fruits are low glycemic. People who battle with their weight often say their favorite fruit is watermelon, that's because its high glycemic. Watermelon is water; sugar and far too little fiber to offset the sugar -- remember G Factor Rules 2 and 3? Most fruits are low, a few are moderate so consult the index. As for cakes, etc. refined foods are out -- plain and simple. If you're a GK 5 and really if you're a GK 4, as well, but type GK 4's may be able to cheat a little without fat gain. Having said that (knowing some will cheat regardless) refined foods are unhealthy even if they don't cause fat gain in some people in some circumstances. Refined flours are unnatural to the human diet and unhealthy for your body. Yes, there

are some recipes that you can keep in the GK zone with them, but I recommend avoiding them all together. Make your choice by consulting the tables, but make sure you stay in the GK Zone.

Question: What if I don't like these choices?
Answer: The menus listed in this book are simply there to give you some guidelines and ideas. Follow the principles I have given you for getting into the GK zone and you will do great!

The suggestions that follow are just that, suggestions. Many people find it difficult to plan their meals with a new concept. With this in mind, below are many suggestions that can help you build a framework for your future eating habits and demonstrate that you will have an amazing variety of choices while you are improving health and getting that excess body fat off your body. I have deliberately been redundant in some areas to reinforce the concepts.

Remember the concept of timing your food intake? It is essential that you keep your blood sugar at normal levels and this is why I have so many snacks scheduled. If your blood sugar stays normal, you will have the main cause of appetite controlled and you will burn stored fat until you reach your body's metabolic weight set point. After that, it will help you maintain weight at a healthy level.

I have added frequent recommendations for additional fiber to the daily suggested menus. Fiber not only helps us feel full, but we get far too little of it in our daily modern diet to be truly healthy. Colon health is largely dependent on fiber intake.

These suggestions are just that, suggestions. Use these ideas to help guide you in future meal planning. These have already been calculated for the glycemic, index, calories, and fat grams. **Bon Appetit!**

Suggested Menus
Day 1

Morning:
  8 oz. Low glycemic meal replacement drink. Meal replacement drinks are designed to help maintain weight or take weight off, depending on how they are used.
  Optional: Additional fiber can be added for thickness and to assist with a feeling of fullness. Protein in excess can contribute to weight gain in some people that is why protein drinks are used to increase mass on

body builders. Some people, however, who are hypoglycemic (low blood sugar) may want to experiment with adding some additional protein.

Mid morning snack:
Hard-boiled egg (no salt, it increases appetite)
8 oz. of water
Optional: Additional glucomannan or pectin fiber can be added to your water to assist with a feeling of fullness.

Lunch:
Salad of your choice
Suggestion: Caesar, Greek, Chicken Caesar or Petite Chef
8 oz. of water with 1/2 lemon squeezed in
Optional: Additional glucomannan or pectin fiber can be added for thickness and to assist with a feeling of fullness.
Note: the best salad dressing is extra virgin olive oil. For some, that seems boring but it's the healthiest, and the EFA's have a minor assist for fat burn. A good olive oil can have tremendous flavor!

Afternoon snack:
8 oz. Low glycemic meal replacement drink
Optional: Additional fiber can be added for thickness and to assist with a feeling of fullness. Protein in excess can contribute to weight gain in some people that is why protein drinks are used to increase mass on body builders. Some people, however, who are hypoglycemic (low blood sugar) may want to experiment with adding some additional protein.
Six almonds, cashews, pecans, or 1 oz. of raw or toasted seeds. Almonds are the best choice.

Dinner:
Grilled, baked, or roasted chicken breast w/rosemary, spinach salad, wild brown rice
8 oz. of water
Optional: Additional glucomannan or pectin fiber can be added to assist with a feeling of fullness.

Evening snack:
1/2 cup strawberries or blueberries (no syrup) with plain regular or fat free yogurt for dipping - variation add nuts. **Note:** Natural organic

yogurt would be the best choice.

Sweeteners: Where sweeteners are required use Xylitol, it is low glycemic, natural and, tastes great.

8 oz. of water

Day 2

Morning:

8 oz. Low glycemic meal replacement drink. Meal replacement drinks are designed to help maintain weight or take weight off, depending on how they are used.

Optional: Additional fiber can be added for thickness and to assist with a feeling of fullness. Protein in excess can contribute to weight gain in some people that is why protein drinks are used to increase mass on body builders. Some people, however, who are hypoglycemic (low blood sugar) may want to experiment with adding some additional protein.

Mid morning snack:

1/2 cup cottage cheese with 8-10 almonds, cashews or pecans

8 oz. of water

Optional: Additional glucomannan or pectin fiber can be added for thickness and to assist with a feeling of fullness.

Lunch:

Egg salad with tomato. After the first fourteen days on the diet, you can add in low glycemic bread to make an egg salad sandwich.

8 oz. of water with 1/2 lemon squeezed in

Optional: Additional glucomannan or pectin fiber can be added for thickness and to assist with a feeling of fullness.

Afternoon snack:

8 oz. Low glycemic meal replacement drink

Optional: Additional fiber can be added for thickness and to assist with a feeling of fullness. Protein in excess can contribute to weight gain in some people that is why protein drinks are used to increase mass on body builders. Some people, however, who are hypoglycemic (low blood sugar) may want to experiment with adding some additional protein.

8-10 almonds, cashews, pecans, or 1 oz. of seeds

Dinner:
>   Grilled/broiled steak (6 oz.) lightly steamed broccoli or wok fried, sweet
>   potato w/real butter, no brown sugar
>   8 oz. of water
>   **Optional:** Additional glucomannan or pectin fiber can be added for
>   thickness and to assist with a feeling of fullness.

Evening snack:
>   1/2 cup of fat free or low fat yogurt with 8-10 almonds, cashews or
>   pecans
>   8 oz. of water
>   **Optional:** Additional glucomannan or pectin fiber can be added for
>   thickness and to assist with a feeling of fullness.

Day 3

Morning:
>   8 oz. Low glycemic meal replacement drink
>   Meal replacement drinks are designed to help maintain weight or take
>   weight off, depending on how they are used.
>   **Optional:** Additional fiber can be added for thickness and to assist with
>   a feeling of fullness. Protein in excess can contribute to weight gain in
>   some people that is why protein drinks are used to increase mass on
>   body builders. Some people however, who are hypoglycemic (low blood
>   sugar) may want to experiment with adding some additional protein.

Mid morning snack:
>   Celery sticks stuffed with peanut butter or cream cheese
>   8 oz. of water.
>   **Optional:** Additional glucomannan or pectin fiber can be added for
>   thickness and to assist with a feeling of fullness.

Lunch:
>   4-6 oz. Grilled, blackened or broiled fish, garden salad vinaigrette dress-
>   ing w/nuts
>   8 oz. of water with 1/2 lemon squeezed in
>   **Optional:** Additional glucomannan or pectin fiber can be added for
>   thickness and to assist with a feeling of fullness.

Afternoon snack:

>8 oz. Low glycemic meal replacement drink
>**Optional:** Additional fiber can be added for thickness and to assist with a feeling of fullness. Protein in excess can contribute to weight gain in some people that is why protein drinks are used to increase mass on body builders. Some people, however, who are hypoglycemic (low blood sugar) may want to experiment with adding some additional protein.
>6-10 almonds, cashews, pecans, or 1 oz. of seeds

Dinner:

>Roasted chicken breast, 3 bean salad, mashed cauliflower (white potato substitute) w/garlic and real butter
>8 oz. of water
>**Optional:** Additional glucomannan or pectin fiber can be added for thickness and to assist with a feeling of fullness.

Evening snack:

>1/2 cup of cottage cheese. Note, taking your omegas with cottage cheese is more effective if you use plant source omegas. As little as one ounce of cottage cheese can make a difference. If you avoid dairy, use a free form amino acid capsule called cysteine instead. You will achieve the same results.
>8 oz. of water
>**Optional:** Additional glucomannan or pectin fiber can be added for thickness and to assist with a feeling of fullness.

Day 4

Morning:

>8 oz. Low glycemic meal replacement drink
>Meal replacement drinks are designed to help maintain weight or take weight off, depending on how they are used.
>**Optional:** Additional fiber can be added for thickness and to assist with a feeling of fullness. Protein in excess can contribute to weight gain in some people that is why protein drinks are used to increase mass on body builders. Some people however, who are hypoglycemic (low blood sugar) may want to experiment with adding some additional protein.

Mid morning snack:

>Hard-boiled egg (no salt, it increases appetite)

8 oz. of water
Optional: Additional glucomannan or pectin fiber can be added for thickness and to assist with a feeling of fullness.

Lunch:
Caesar with grilled chicken breast or salad of your choice such as petite Cobb or chef salad, no croutons
8 oz. of water with 1/2 lemon squeezed in
Optional: Additional glucomannan or pectin fiber can be added for thickness and to assist with a feeling of fullness.

Afternoon snack:
8 oz. Low glycemic meal replacement drink
Optional: Additional fiber can be added for thickness and to assist with a feeling of fullness. Protein in excess can contribute to weight gain in some people that is why protein drinks are used to increase mass on body builders. Some people, however, who are hypoglycemic (low blood sugar) may want to experiment with adding some additional protein.
6-10 almonds, cashews, pecans, or 1 oz. of seeds

Dinner:
Hamburger (lean, no bun), garden salad with romaine lettuce, no croutons, baked (low sugar, but not artificially sweetened) or black beans. Brands of baked beans that sell the best have the highest levels of sugars in them. Read the labels.
8 oz. of water
Optional: Additional glucomannan or pectin fiber can be added for thickness and to assist with a feeling of fullness.

Evening snack:
1 cup of plain fat-free yogurt with 1/2 cup of fresh berries
8 oz. of water
Optional: Additional glucomannan or pectin fiber can be added for thickness and to assist with a feeling of fullness.

Day 5

Morning:
8 oz. Low glycemic meal replacement drink
Meal replacement drinks are designed to help maintain weight or take

weight off, depending on how they are used.

Optional: Additional fiber can be added for thickness and to assist with a feeling of fullness. Protein in excess can contribute to weight gain in some people that is why protein drinks are used to increase mass on body builders. Some people, however, who are hypoglycemic (low blood sugar) may want to experiment with adding some additional protein.

Mid morning snack:
    1 oz. of fat free cheese
    8 oz. of vegetable cocktail juice
    Optional: Additional glucomannan or pectin fiber can be added for thickness and to assist with a feeling of fullness.

Lunch:
    Ground sirloin burger (no bun), 1 oz. fat-free cheese, small garden salad w/vinaigrette dressing
    8 oz. of water with 1/2 lemon squeezed in
    Optional: Additional glucomannan or pectin fiber can be added for thickness and to assist with a feeling of fullness.

Afternoon snack:
    8 oz. Low glycemic meal replacement drink
    Optional: Additional fiber can be added for thickness and to assist with a feeling of fullness. Protein in excess can contribute to weight gain in some people that is why protein drinks are used to increase mass on body builders. Some people, however, who are hypoglycemic (low blood sugar) may want to experiment with adding some additional protein.
    6-10 almonds, cashews, pecans, or 1 oz. of seeds

Dinner:
    Pork loin w/ sauerkraut, steamed zucchini, mixed green salad w/ olive oil and vinegar dressing
    8 oz. of water
    Optional: Additional glucomannan or pectin fiber can be added for thickness and to assist with a feeling of fullness.

Evening snack:
    1/2 cup strawberries with plain fat-free yogurt for dipping - variation add nuts

8 oz. of water
Optional: Additional glucomannan or pectin fiber can be added for thickness and to assist with a feeling of fullness.

Day 6

Morning
2 Egg omelet with veggie strips (peppers, onions, mushrooms) turkey sausage patty, 8 oz. of vegetable cocktail juice
Optional: Additional glucomannan or pectin fiber can be added for thickness and to assist with a feeling of fullness.

Mid morning snack:
1 cup fat-free or low fat plain yogurt
For variation, add 1 oz. of nuts & seeds.
8 oz. of water
Optional: Additional glucomannan or pectin fiber can be added for thickness and to assist with a feeling of fullness.

Lunch:
8 oz. Low glycemic meal replacement drink
Add 2 tablespoons of plain/vanilla yogurt
Optional: Additional glucomannan or pectin fiber can be added for thickness and to assist with a feeling of fullness. Glucomannan simply gels clear and is both tasteless and odorless and pectin adds a faint citrus accent.

Afternoon snack:
Small apple
6-10 almonds, cashews, pecans, or 1 oz. of seeds
8 oz. of water
Optional: Additional glucomannan or pectin fiber can be added for thickness and to assist with a feeling of fullness.

Dinner:
Broiled or grilled flank steak, (6 oz.) mixed green salad w/ olive oil and vinegar or vinaigrette dressing, 8 oz. of water
Optional: Additional glucomannan or pectin fiber can be added for thickness and to assist with a feeling of fullness.

Evening snack:
1/2 cup of fruit, can add fat free yogurt or sour cream for dipping

8 oz. of water
Optional: Additional glucomannan or pectin fiber can be added for thickness and to assist with a feeling of fullness.

Day 7

Morning:
> 2 Eggs, 1 oz. of fat-free cheese
> 8 oz. of vegetable cocktail juice
> **Optional:** Additional glucomannan or pectin fiber can be added for thickness and to assist with a feeling of fullness.

Mid morning snack:
> Celery sticks stuffed with peanut butter or cream cheese
> 8 oz. of water
> **Optional:** Additional glucomannan or pectin fiber can be added for thickness and to assist with a feeling of fullness.

Lunch:
> 8 oz. Low glycemic meal replacement drink
> **Optional:** Additional fiber can be added for thickness and to assist with a feeling of fullness. Protein in excess can contribute to weight gain in some people that is why protein drinks are used to increase mass on body builders. Some people, however, who are hypoglycemic (low blood sugar) may want to experiment with adding some additional protein.
> 6-10 almonds, cashews, pecans, or 1 oz. of seeds

Afternoon snack:
> Piece of fresh low G fruit
> 6-10 almonds, cashews, pecans, or 1 oz. of seeds
> 8 oz. of water
> **Optional:** Additional glucomannan or pectin fiber can be added for thickness and to assist with a feeling of fullness.

Dinner:
> Grilled, baked/broiled herb covered chicken breast, cucumber salad, wok fried or steamed green beans, 8 oz. of water
> **Optional:** Additional glucomannan or pectin fiber can be added for thickness and to assist with a feeling of fullness.

Evening snack:

Low glycemic meal replacement drink as **ice cream!** Use a double portion of meal replacement powder with 4 ounces of milk or thicken to suit your taste, but do not increase meal replacement powder beyond two servings. Blend thoroughly. Mix with fine ice chips if you choose. The higher the fat content of the milk the thicker the ice cream. Mix to taste, but remember although fat is zero glycemic, too much fat will lead to health issues, so consider this carefully when making your low glycemic ice cream treat. My recommendation is low fat milk. There are people who have been on my diet for many years successfully and use this particular treat daily. Refer to my information on metabolic types to help you decide.

Day 8

Morning:

8 oz. Low glycemic meal replacement drink

Meal replacement drinks are designed to help maintain weight or take weight off, depending on how they are used.

Optional: Additional fiber can be added for thickness and to assist with a feeling of fullness. Protein in excess can contribute to weight gain in some people that is why protein drinks are used to increase mass on body builders. Some people, however, who are hypoglycemic (low blood sugar) may want to experiment with adding some additional protein.

Mid morning snack:

Hardboiled egg (no salt it increases appetite)

8 oz. of water

Optional: Additional glucomannan or pectin fiber can be added for thickness and to assist with a feeling of fullness.

Lunch:

3 Turkey rollups, 1 oz. of cheese

8 oz. of water with 1/2 lemon squeezed in

Optional: Additional glucomannan or pectin fiber can be added for thickness and to assist with a feeling of fullness.

Afternoon snack:

8 oz. Low glycemic meal replacement drink

Meal replacement drinks are designed to help maintain weight or take weight off, depending on how they are used.

Optional: Additional fiber can be added for thickness and to assist with a feeling of fullness. Protein in excess can contribute to weight gain in some people that is why protein drinks are used to increase mass on body builders. Some people, however, who are hypoglycemic (low blood sugar) may want to experiment with adding some additional protein.

6 – 10 almonds, pecans, cashews, or 1 oz. of seeds

Dinner:

Ground turkey meatloaf, steamed or wok-fried broccoli & pepper strips, mixed green salad w/ olive oil and vinaigrette dressing, 8 oz. of water
Optional: Additional glucomannan or pectin fiber can be added for thickness and to assist with a feeling of fullness.

Evening snack:

1/2 cup cottage cheese
8 oz. of water
Optional: Additional glucomannan or pectin fiber can be added for thickness and to assist with a feeling of fullness.

Day 9

Morning:

8 oz. Low glycemic meal replacement drink
Meal replacement drinks are designed to help maintain weight or take weight off depending on how they are used. Considering the total numbers of this days menu you could add 2 ounces plain regular yogurt to enhance your low G drink.
Optional: Additional fiber can be added for thickness and to assist with a feeling of fullness. Protein in excess can contribute to weight gain in some people that is why protein drinks are used to increase mass on body builders. Some people, however, who are hypoglycemic (low blood sugar) may want to experiment with adding some additional protein.

Mid morning snack:

1/2 cup plain fat free or low fat yogurt and some unsweetened granola for a crunchy taste and the fiber helps to slow the index.
8 oz. of water
Optional: Additional glucomannan or pectin fiber can be added for thickness and to assist with a feeling of fullness.

Lunch:
>   Tuna or egg salad, w/ cherry tomatoes
>   8 oz. of water with 1/2 lemon squeezed in
>   **Optional:** Additional glucomannan or pectin fiber can be added for
>   thickness and to assist with a feeling of fullness.

Afternoon snack:
>   8 oz. Low glycemic meal replacement drink
>   Meal replacement drinks are designed to help maintain weight or take
>   weight off depending on how they are used.
>   **Optional:** Additional fiber can be added for thickness and to assist with
>   a feeling of fullness. Protein in excess can contribute to weight gain in
>   some people that is why protein drinks are used to increase mass on
>   body builders. Some people, however, who are hypoglycemic (low
>   blood sugar) may want to experiment with adding some additional
>   protein.
>   6 – 10 almonds, pecans, cashews, or 1 oz. of seeds

Dinner:
>   Grilled/broiled chicken breast w/balsamic marinade, mashed cauliflower,
>   tomato and mozzarella salad, 8 oz. of water
>   **Optional:** Additional glucomannan or pectin fiber can be added for
>   thickness and to assist with a feeling of fullness.

Evening snack:
>   1/2 cup of fruit, can add fat free yogurt or sour cream for dipping
>   8 oz. of water
>   **Optional:** Additional glucomannan or pectin fiber can be added for
>   thickness and to assist with a feeling of fullness.

Day 10

Morning:
>   8 oz. Low glycemic meal replacement drink
>   Meal replacement drinks are designed to help maintain weight or take
>   weight off, depending on how they are used.
>   **Optional:** Additional fiber can be added for thickness and to assist with
>   a feeling of fullness. Protein in excess can contribute to weight gain in
>   some people that is why protein drinks are used to increase mass on
>   body builders. Some people, however, who are hypoglycemic (low

blood sugar) may want to experiment with adding some additional protein.

Mid morning snack:
Celery sticks stuffed with fresh peanut butter or cream cheese
8 oz. of water
Optional: Additional glucomannan or pectin fiber can be added for thickness and to assist with a feeling of fullness.

Lunch:
Slice of turkey meatloaf, mixed green salad with balsamic dressing
8 oz. of water
Optional: Additional glucomannan or pectin fiber can be added for thickness and to assist with a feeling of fullness.

Afternoon snack:
8 oz. Low glycemic meal replacement drink
Meal replacement drinks are designed to help maintain weight or take weight off, depending on how they are used.
Optional: Additional fiber can be added for thickness and to assist with a feeling of fullness. Protein in excess can contribute to weight gain in some people that is why protein drinks are used to increase mass on body builders. Some people, however, who are hypoglycemic (low blood sugar) may want to experiment with adding some additional protein.
6 – 10 almonds, pecans, cashews or 1 oz. of seeds

Dinner:
Grilled/broiled fish of your choice, cucumber salad, steamed green beans
8 oz. of water
Optional: Additional glucomannan or pectin fiber can be added for thickness and to assist with a feeling of fullness.

Evening snack:
1/2 cup of plain fat free yogurt w/ fresh berries
8 oz. of water
Optional: Additional glucomannan or pectin fiber can be added for thickness and to assist with a feeling of fullness.
Consult the G Factor Food index for further planning.

Day 11

Morning:
> 8 oz. Low glycemic meal replacement drink
> **Optional:** Additional fiber can be added for thickness and to assist with a feeling of fullness. Protein in excess can contribute to weight gain in some people that is why protein drinks are used to increase mass on body builders. Some people, however, who are hypoglycemic (low blood sugar) may want to experiment with adding some additional protein.

Mid morning snack:
> Low glycemic fruit or chocolate bar or 1 oz. of low fat cheese or 6-10 almonds
> 12 oz. of water
> **Optional:** Additional glucomannan or pectin fiber can be added for thickness and to assist with a feeling of fullness.

Lunch:
> Greek Garbanzo Bean Salad with Feta cheese
> 12 oz. of water with 1/2 lemon squeezed in
> **Optional:** Additional glucomannan or pectin fiber can be added for thickness and to assist with a feeling of fullness.

Afternoon snack:
> 8 oz. Low glycemic meal replacement drink
> **Optional:** Additional fiber can be added for thickness and to assist with a feeling of fullness. Protein in excess can contribute to weight gain in some people that is why protein drinks are used to increase mass on body builders. Some people, however, who are hypoglycemic (low blood sugar) may want to experiment with adding some additional protein.
> 6-10 almonds, pecans or 1 oz. of seeds

Dinner:
> Grilled, baked/broiled pork lion chops, black bean salad, steamed broccoli,
> 12 oz. of water
> **Optional:** Additional glucomannan or pectin fiber can be added for thickness and to assist with a feeling of fullness.

Evening snack:

    Low glycemic meal replacement drink as ice cream! Use a double portion of meal replacement powder with 4 ounces of milk or thicken to suit your taste, but do not increase meal replacement powder beyond two servings. Blend thoroughly. Mix with fine ice chips if you choose.

Day 12

Morning:

    8 oz. Low glycemic meal replacement drink.

    Optional: Additional fiber can be added for thickness and to assist with a feeling of fullness. Protein in excess can contribute to weight gain in some people that is why protein drinks are used to increase mass on body builders. Some people, however, who are hypoglycemic (low blood sugar) may want to experiment with adding some additional protein.

Mid morning snack:

    1/2 cup cottage cheese with 8-10 almonds, or pecans

    12 oz. of water

    Optional: Additional glucomannan or pectin fiber can be added for thickness and to assist with a feeling of fullness.

Lunch:

    Black Bean salad (left over from dinner)

    12 oz. of water with 1/2 lemon squeezed in

    Optional: Additional glucomannan or pectin fiber can be added for thickness and to assist with a feeling of fullness.

Afternoon snack:

    8 oz. Low glycemic meal replacement drink

    Optional: Additional fiber can be added for thickness and to assist with a feeling of fullness. Protein in excess can contribute to weight gain in some people that is why protein drinks are used to increase mass on body builders. Some people however who are hypoglycemic (low blood sugar) may want to experiment with adding some additional protein.

    8-10 almonds, cashews, pecans or 1 oz. of seeds

Dinner:

    Chicken veggie stir-fry with spinach salad and vinaigrette or olive oil & vinegar dressing

12 oz. of water
Optional: Additional glucomannan or pectin fiber can be added for thickness and to assist with a feeling of fullness.

Evening snack:
1/2 cup of fat free or low fat yogurt with 8-10 almonds or pecans
12 oz. of water
Optional: Additional glucomannan or pectin fiber can be added for thickness and to assist with a feeling of fullness.

Day 13

Morning:
Cheese and veggie frittata with Canadian bacon slices
8 oz. of vegetable cocktail juice
Optional: Additional fiber can be added for thickness and to assist with a feeling of fullness. Protein in excess can contribute to weight gain in some people that is why protein drinks are used to increase mass on body builders. Some people, however, who are hypoglycemic (low blood sugar) may want to experiment with adding some additional protein.

Mid morning snack:
Celery sticks stuffed with fresh peanut butter or cream cheese
12 oz. of water.
Optional: Additional glucomannan or pectin fiber can be added for thickness and to assist with a feeling of fullness.

Lunch:
8 oz. Low glycemic meal replacement drink
Optional: Additional fiber can be added for thickness and to assist with a feeling of fullness. Protein in excess can contribute to weight gain in some people that is why protein drinks are used to increase mass on body builders. Some people, however, who are hypoglycemic (low blood sugar) may want to experiment with adding some additional protein.

Afternoon snack:
Piece of fresh fruit on green list, or
8-10 almonds, pecans or 1 oz. of seeds
12 oz. of water

Optional: Additional glucomannan or pectin fiber can be added for thickness and to assist with a feeling of fullness.

Dinner:
Pork loin roast, (any meat may be substituted for pork) broccoli rabe, mashed navy beans with butter
12 oz. of water
Optional: Additional glucomannan or pectin fiber can be added for thickness and to assist with a feeling of fullness.

Evening snack:
Low glycemic fruit & yogurt or chocolate bar.
12 oz. of water
Optional: Additional glucomannan or pectin fiber can be added for thickness and to assist with a feeling of fullness.

Day 14

Morning:
2 Eggs, 1 oz. of fat free cheese
12 oz. of vegetable cocktail juice
Optional: Additional glucomannan or pectin fiber can be added for thickness and to assist with a feeling of fullness.

Mid morning snack:
2 turkey roll ups
12 oz. of water
Optional: Additional glucomannan or pectin fiber can be added for thickness and to assist with a feeling of fullness.

Lunch:
8 oz. Low glycemic meal replacement drink
Optional: Additional fiber can be added for thickness and to assist with a feeling of fullness. Protein in excess can contribute to weight gain in some people that is why protein drinks are used to increase mass on body builders. Some people, however, who are hypoglycemic (low blood sugar) may want to experiment with adding some additional protein.

Afternoon snack:
    Piece of fresh fruit on green list
    8-10 almonds, cashews, pecans or 1 oz. of seeds
    12 oz. of water with 1/2 lemon squeezed in
    Optional: Additional glucomannan or pectin fiber can be added for thickness and to assist with a feeling of fullness.

Dinner:
    Roasted Turkey breast, zucchini with dill, Mediterranean kale and tomato salad
    12 oz. of water
    Optional: Additional glucomannan or pectin fiber can be added for thickness and to assist with a feeling of fullness.

Evening snack:
    Low glycemic meal replacement drink as ice cream! Use a double portion of meal replacement powder with 4 ounces of milk or thicken to suit your taste, but do not increase meal replacement powder beyond two servings. Blend thoroughly. Mix with fine ice chips if you choose. 12 oz. of water.

Suggested recipes

Three bean salad

6 oz. of thin green beans ends, trimmed, cut in 1 1/2" lengths
12 oz. of frozen lima beans
One 16 oz. can of red kidney beans, drained and rinsed
shallots, sliced for garnish

Dressing
6 tablespoons virgin olive oil
1 1/2 to 2 tablespoons of red wine vinegar (can use Balsamic)
2 small shallots, finely chopped
Salt & black pepper to taste

Cook green beans in boiling water for 5 minutes and drain. Cook lima beans according to package directions, drain. In a bowl combine all beans. Prepare dressing and pour over beans tossing until coated. Garnish with shallot rings. Cover and refrigerate until ready to serve.

Tomato & Mozzarella salad

2 large beef steak tomatoes, sliced
6 oz. fat free mozzarella sliced
1 small red onion sliced
1/4 cup Balsamic vinegar
1 tablespoon of fresh basil
Salt & pepper to taste
1 tablespoon pine nuts

Arrange tomato and cheese slices on a plate (can be done on 4 salad plates) Top with onion rings. Season with S&P to taste, drizzle balsamic vinegar, sprinkle with basil and pine nuts. For variation sprinkle 1/4 cup of extra virgin olive oil and try different seasoning combinations such as dill or cilantro.

Yogurt dressing

2/3 cup of plain fat-free yogurt
2 tablespoons of lemon juice
1 teaspoon of Dijon style mustard
1 teaspoon of honey
Salt & pepper to taste

In a bowl whisk all ingredients until smooth and creamy. Refrigerate 30 minutes before using.

Variations:
Add 2 tablespoons of chopped fresh or dried herbs such as tarragon, mint, parsley, chives or garlic. Try combinations to suit your salad or veggies. You may also wish to add some phytonutrient powder to your mix for enhanced flavor and nutrition. This can be a great substitute for mayo.

Mediterranean Spinach

4 medium bunches fresh spinach
1/2 TBS lemon juice
1/2 TBS balsamic vinegar
2 medium cloves fresh garlic, pressed
1 TBS extra virgin olive oil
salt & cracked black pepper to taste

Bring lightly salted water to a rapid boil in a large pot. Cut stems off spinach leaves and clean well. This can be done easily by leaving spinach bundled and cutting off stems all at once. **Rinse spinach leaves very well as they often contain a lot of soil.** Cook spinach in simmering water for 2 minutes.

Drain and press out excess water. Toss in rest of ingredients and serve. Toss spinach with dressing just before you are ready to serve.

Mediterranean Kale

2 medium bunches kale, chopped about 12 cups
2 TBS lemon juice
1 tsp soy sauce
3 medium cloves garlic, pressed
extra virgin olive oil to taste
salt & black pepper to taste
Bring lightly salted water to a boil in a steamer with a tight fitting lid. The salt helps to enhance flavor and color of vegetables. While water is coming to a boil, fold each kale leaf in half and pull or cut out stem. Chop leaf and rinse in colander. When water comes to a boil add kale to steamer basket and cover. Steam for 8 minutes.
Toss with rest of ingredients and serve

Baked Herb Chicken

2 medium cloves of garlic chopped or pressed
1 tablespoon of lemon juice
2 tsp of chopped fresh sage
2 tsp of chopped fresh thyme
2 tsp of chopped fresh rosemary
1/4 cup chicken broth
4 Boneless/skinless chicken breasts (pounded if desired)
Salt & pepper to taste

Mix together first 6 ingredients in a saucepan sauté for 4-5 minutes on low heat. Place chicken breasts in an oven safe dish. Sprinkle with salt and pepper, then pour or brush herb mixture over each breast. Bake for 25 - 30 minutes in 350-degree oven. Ovens vary on efficiency, some ovens may require more time. Make sure the chicken is thoroughly cooked.

Black Bean Salad

1 15 oz. can of black beans, drained & rinsed
8 cherry or grape tomatoes
1/2 cup of minced onions
2 medium cloves of garlic chopped or pressed
1/2 cup of diced red bell peppers (can use yellow)
1/4 cup chopped fresh cilantro
2 tbs. extra virgin olive oil
3 tbs. fresh lemon juice
salt & pepper to taste

Mix all ingredients and chill and serve. This can be kept for several days and gets better as the flavors marinate together. Variation: add sunflower, flax or chopped pumpkin seeds.

Greek Garbanzo Bean salad

1 15 oz. can of garbanzo beans, drained & rinsed
2/3 cup minced scallion
3 medium cloves of garlic chopped or pressed
1 medium tomato, seeds removed and chopped

2 stalks of celery, chopped medium pieces
3 tbs. fresh lemon juice
2 & 1/2 tbs. chopped fresh mint
3 tbs. chopped fresh parsley
3 tbs. virgin olive oil
4 - 6 oz. of Feta cheese (optional)
1 small head of romaine or other red leafed lettuce, washed and dried
salt & pepper to taste

Combine all ingredients except lettuce and cheese in a bowl. Tear leaves of lettuce into strips and place on plates. Place salad mixture on top, sprinkle with cheese and serve.

Mashed Navy Beans

2 cans of navy beans, drained
1 medium onion chopped
6 cloves of garlic chopped
1 tsp chopped fresh rosemary
2 + 1 tbs. vegetable broth
Salt and pepper to taste

Heat 1 tbs. of vegetable broth over medium to low heat. Add onions and sauté for 5 minutes then add garlic. Sauté for one more minute. Add the rest of the broth, beans and rosemary; continue heating for 5 minutes.

Remove from heat and puree in a blender or chopper until smooth. You should add gradually and scrape sides. Salt & Pepper to taste

Cheese & veggie Frittata

1 Cup Broccoli Florets
3/4 Cup Sliced Fresh Mushroom
2 Green Onions — finely chopped
1 Tablespoon Butter
1 Cup Cubed Fully Cooked turkey or chicken breast (optional)
8 Eggs
1/4 Cup Water
1/4 Cup Dijon Mustard
1/2 Teaspoon Italian Seasoning
1/4 Teaspoon Garlic Salt

1 1/2 Cups (6 ounces) Shredded Cheddar Cheese

1/2 Cup Chopped Tomatoes

In a skillet, sauté the broccoli, mushrooms and onions in butter until tender. Add meat (optional); heat through. Remove from the heat and keep warm. In a mixing bowl, beat eggs, water, mustard, Italian seasoning and garlic salt until foamy. Stir in cheese, tomatoes and broccoli mixture. Pour into a greased shallow 1-1/2 quart baking dish. Bake at 375 degrees F. for 22-27 minutes or until a knife inserted in the center comes out clean. Yields 4-6 servings. Consider adding a great salad and make this an easy dinner or lunch.

Chapter 10
The truth about exercise and diet, it's not what you think

I have heard every excuse you can think of regarding exercise. If you choose not to exercise, it's a choice. Almost no one has an excuse to avoid exercise every-day of their lives.

Here are some of my favorites
- I don't have time
- I am too tired
- I travel too much in my job
- I can't afford a gym membership or home equipment

I am going to address those excuses, but to make it simple those are reasons not excuses.

In 2005, I was on the road 310 days out of 365. Do you travel more than me?

My typical day is an early morning trip to the airport and flight to cities in any of 10 or more countries. When I arrive at my lecture venue, there are meetings and conference calls that go on all day until the evening lecture, which is near-ly always preceded by a business dinner. After the lecture, that takes at least two hours, I typically answer questions that can go on for hours. When I get to my hotel room, my average day has lasted 14 to 18 hours, sometimes longer. I have had many 20-hour days. In between all that I have to answer e-mails and do research, as well as, write information for a number of publications as part of my job. Are your days busier than mine?

Do you think I'm not tired from my schedule and workload?

You don't need a gym membership. I will give you suggestions for things you can do without equipment right in your home or hotel room.

I prefer to use the word activity rather then exercise because exercise has so many negative connotations. First people think of exercise as unpleasant, as hard work, evil, or something that distracts them from having fun. But any activ-ity can help you in your quest to increase lean body mass, and/or improve body composition. Well I say any activity, obviously would preclude activity such as pushing the buttons on the remote control. But activities should start light or moderate, unless of course you are already very physically active. Of course, it is important to note that you should consult your physician before beginning any exercise program.

An increase in activity can help you burn a small number of calories, but activity in and of itself for the purpose of weight loss, is actually misunderstood. As an example, if you were to run as fast as you could for 30 minutes non-stop, you would burn off the equivalent calories of a bologna sandwich. How many hours can you run non-stop each day? Obviously, exercise is an important component of a complete program, but exercise alone, unless you are very young, and/or have a high metabolism, will not keep the fat off.

What is important about exercise is that it not only improves your cardiovascular health, which is well known, but in addition it helps to tone your muscles, and depending on the exercise you choose, increases lean muscle mass. Going back to our discussion on scale weight or pounds, it is important to note that as you attain a leaner, healthier body, you may actually weigh more. But your total body in terms of the way it looks, in terms of the number of inches, in terms of the clothing that you fit into, will be far more positive. For example, a woman goes from a size 18 dress, to a size 9 dress, but actually increases her body weight in the process, this is a positive thing. So let's not fixate on pounds.

It is important that you warm up before exercise. One of the first big mistakes people make when they begin an exercise program is that they do too much, too quickly. They are impatient for a given result, and don't do appropriate warm-up exercises before they begin the exercise.

Warming up basically consists of stretching your muscles, doing stretches on your legs, arms, and back. Stretching the muscles increases the blood flow to the muscles, which is known as warming up. If you stretch before you begin physical exercise, you will be less sore, with less discomfort from the exercise as a result.

No pain no gain? Is that really true? Well, this truly depends on your short term, as well as long term goals, the condition you're in when you begin, and whether you do it wisely or foolishly. If you begin your program wisely and work your way up to your goal gradually, there should be little or no discomfort. If your planned goal is an extreme one, such as body building, you can still reduce the discomfort suffered by others by doing warm ups, but for some body building, muscle soreness is a given.

Aerobic VS Anaerobic

Another mistake made by many people, particularly women on diets, is to do only aerobic exercise. Aerobic exercise is valuable for your cardiovascular fitness; it will help to burn some small percentage of calories and fat. It will help to light the fire on your metabolism, and help you slowly over take what is known as the weight set point. But it is important that women and men do exercises for toning the muscles as well. As you increase muscle tone, and if you supply sufficient protein in your daily diet, you can also increase some measure of muscle mass. You will find that you burn fat more efficiently with increased muscle mass; burning fat more efficiently is key to keeping the weight off once you have lost it.

This doesn't mean that any male or female needs to become Mr. or Ms. Universe. Simple and light resistance exercise can accomplish your goal for toning, fitness and fat burn.

The first exercise any human ever got was probably walking; it still is one of the best. Exercising the quadriceps, which require the most oxygen and are the large long muscle between your knees and your hips, is by far the most important for cardiovascular fitness and aerobic in general. Walking, running, cycling, dancing, all work nicely for those muscles. Getting more ambitious, boxing, kickboxing, Tae bo and so on also work these muscle. Keeping this simple and 0 cost, walking is great! Yes there are a zillion other methods I have not mentioned, but you get the idea.

Exercise programs can be highly individualized and for many people should be. But in general, it is important to start with a warm up or stretching period. The next step should include walking or cycling. either on a treadmill, sky machine or a bike for at least 11 minutes on a minimum setting, or a pace that is comfortable for you. It is very important that you don't try more than you are capable of at first, but 11 or more minutes should be a first level goal. Remember the old axiom, "slow and steady wins the race". If you do too much, too soon, and your body isn't capable of dealing with it, you will end up quitting your program, and perhaps injuring yourself as well. As you slowly add to the amount of exercise you do each day, you will find that you begin to feel better, more energetic, more alert, and more positive. The better you feel, the easier it will be to increase your activity levels. You'll be surprised, but after a certain point you will enjoy exercising and look forward to it, even feel deprived if you don't do it.

Muscle mass is dense lean and firm. The more muscle you have, the easier it is to keep the fat off and the better you'll feel. If you gear your activity to toning and fitness rather than body building, you will be thinner, leaner, and fit into the clothes you've been looking forward to. Bodybuilding will of course increase your size. It's your choice.

Resistance or anaerobic activity
There seem to be endless devices and machines available for resistance exercise. You have to decide what your goals are. As a male, I wanted to trim the fluffy fat and increase the muscle mass slightly to the point of clear muscle definition of my arms, chest, and shoulders, so I began heavier resistance in those areas. I did not wish to become Mr. Olympia, so my workout was geared accordingly to ensure I get at least 100 grams of protein daily to maintain what I have achieved. Increasing and maintaining muscle requires protein because muscle is approximately 75% water and 25% protein.

The simple no-cost resistance plan
Stretching
Push-ups work
Crunches (not sit ups)

For the more ambitious
Do the above but add the following:
Running in place… start with 11 minutes minimum and gradually add even as little as an extra minute a day until you work your way up to 30 minutes. Remember this is for the ambitious individuals who are in good shape, not beginners. *Your current level of cardiovascular fitness is key so be sure you have your doctors ok before you get too ambitious.*

If you don't like running, try walking in place, but lifting your knees high with each step and do it rapidly, you'll be amazed at the sweat you can work up.
My favorite is shadow boxing (a most wonderful and amazing workout), if you develop a routine of dancing like boxers do in the ring as you shadow box; the cardiovascular workout and fat burn will be very productive and very satisfying!

Do one of the above routines when you get into very good shape. You can and should do all three every day or every other day.

To work muscles for definition and to some extent size or to maintain what you have achieved when you are at a location that has no gym, try finding anything with weight such as a phone book and using it in place of dumbbells. With lighter weight do more repetitions. Also by doing the repetitions very slowly you can get more efficient workouts. You'll be amazed at the results. Curls and extensions, for you experienced veterans can be done easily with any kind of object. When I am going to be in a city one to two full days, I buy a gallon of water and use it for my weights to workout and then drink it to re-hydrate.

A few quick thoughts
Fat cannot become muscle and muscle cannot become fat. They are different cells entirely.

Muscle has memory, so if you have to miss a workout or go for a time without one, your muscles will remember their peak and will want to return there with your help.

More isn't always better.

Injuring yourself will only set you back, so plan your activities wisely.

Exercise program for the beginner at a glance
Remember to check with your physician to determine at which level you should start, but in general beginners should start as follows.

Before you begin any exercise, make sure you stretch those muscles. If you have never stretched them before or haven't in a long time, start with very short easy stretches. Walking is a good way to start.

Stretching (to warm up the muscles)
Walking at a normal pace for a comfortable distance
Each day try to increase your distance a bit and your pace, but stay in the comfort zone at first.
Crunches, start slow, don't push too hard at first, gradually you will strengthen your back and abdominal muscles. Increase between 1-5 crunches if you can every other day.
Push-ups definitely for males but not all females will want to do this one. In the U.S. the current fad is for women to have somewhat muscular arms, but this is not the case in almost any other country. Some toning of the muscles is desirable and beneficial, but experts will continue to debate how healthy it is for women to have significant muscle bulk. Without extraordinary effort, men are naturally more muscular than women. This is because testosterone encourages the production and retention of muscle. Men are testosterone primary.

Estrogen encourages the deposition and retention of fat and women are estrogen primary. In fact, on average, a female has to work about 300% harder than a male to achieve the same results. It is therefore, not the natural state of a women's body to be muscular. I am not making a value judgment, nor expressing my likes or dislikes, simply expressing the facts. Resistance exercise does help to increase bone mass so women do need to do some resistance -- the question is, what level? Once again, life is full of choices.

Bottom line with resistance exercise is your muscles will enjoy becoming stronger and tighter and so will you. Don't over do it, injury never helps.

The type and amounts of exercise are almost endless, but what you have just read is enough to get you started

The better you feel, the more **active** you'll want to be naturally. Many will want to begin fitness programs as they feel better, but we want to start with simple (positive) fun activity and the rest will come naturally.

Closing Comments

I have not come up with a way to break the laws of physics and human physiology. That simply cannot be done with any product or system that exists, pharmaceutical or otherwise. This system requires healthy eating, behavior modification, and increased activity.

Behavior modification includes changes in your eating habits. High G foods are bad for you... end of story. They are the root of the problem for the vast majority of people who are overweight. High G foods are life threatening in the long run, due to pancreatic stress and the contribution to obesity. Excess body and blood fats contribute to heart disease, stroke, some cancers and diabetes. High G foods cause the liver to produce those blood fats. So it is a vitally important health issue to have everyone minimize, or preferably eliminate, high G foods from their lives. As we entered the 21st century, it was reported that the sale of oversize coffins is up 20%. Overweight bodies are more prone to disease and premature death.

More than 1/3 of American's get **0** exercise other than walking to the refrigerator or pushing the button on the remote control! Another 25% get almost no exercise. If you're not being active, yet you need to start.

After more than 20 years as a health care practitioner, I can tell you that one of the principle reasons for the lack of physical "activity" is that people don't have enough energy. They want to come home, eat high glycemic foods while watching TV to bring up their energy and feel a little better (temporarily) before bed. When blood sugar levels dropped in the afternoon, fatigue set in and the craving for high glycemic snacks and stimulants became over-whelming, candy, pastries, coffee, cola's etc.

This is a vicious cycle that reduces quality of life and life spans. You can make a difference by making the right choices. You can be lean, healthy and vigorous. You can prevent heart disease and diabetes. You can increase your life potential and life span. You can not only look better but also enjoy a tremendous sense of well-being. You now know what to do.

Life is full of choices…I hope you choose wisely.

The Genetic Key Diet

Bibliography

1. Renaud, Jean, Insulin and Obesity, Diabetologia 1979, 133-138

2. Jenkins, David J.A., et al. "Glycemic Index of Foods: a Physiological Basis for Carbohydrate Exchange." *The American Journal of Clinical Nutrition*, Vol. 34, March 1981, pp. 362-366.

3. Salmerón, Jorge, et al. "Dietary Fiber, Glycemic Load, and Risk of Non-insulin-dependent Diabetes Mellitus in Women." *The Journal of the American Medical Association*, Vol. 277, February 12, 1997, pp. 472-477.

4. Willett, Walter C. *Eat, Drink, and Be Healthy: The Harvard Medical School Guide to Healthy Eating.* New York: Simon & Schuster Source, 2001.

5. Jenkins DJA, Wolever TMS, Kalmusky J, et al Low Glycemic index carbohydrate foods in the management of hyperlipidemia. American Journal of Clinical Nutrition 1985; 45:604-617

6. Frost G, Wilding GPH, Beecham J, advice based o the glycemic index improves dietary profile and metabolic control I type 2 diabetic patients. Diabetic Medicine 1994; 11: 397-401

7. Glycemic load, diet, and health. *Harv Womens Health Watch.* 2001; 8: 1-2.
8. At year's end: diet, glycemic index, and the food pyramid. *Harv Womens Health Watch.* 2000 Dec; 8: 1-2.

9. Watters K;Blaisdell G 4;. Reduction of glycemic and lipid levels in db/db diabetic mice by psyllium plant fiber. *Diabetes.* 1989 Dec; 38: 1528-1533.

10. Eidenier, H., et al, A Manual for Metabolic/Nutritional Evaluation of the SMA/25, CBC w/Differential and Related Tests, 1995 Rev 1: 20-25

11. Nugent GK1; Ramberg J;. Reassessing the need for dietary supplements for America's children. GlycoScience & Nutrition. 2001 Apr 27;2: 1-7

12. Mogher,K., et al, Diabetes Epidemic and the Thrifty Gene, IMAJ 2002;4:720±721, Diabetes Center and Department of Internal Medicine, Hadassah University Hospital, Jerusalem, Israel

13. Jeppesen, J., Schaaf, G 4., Jones, C., Zhou, MY., Chen, YD., Reaven, RD. Effects of low-fat, high-carbohydrate diets on risk factors for ischemic heart disease in postmenopausal women [published erratum appears in Am J Clin Nutr 1997 Aug;66(2):437] Department of Medicine, Stanford University School of Medicine, CA, USA.

14. Anders Green [1*], Niels Christian Hirsch [2], Stig Krøger Pramming [3] **The changing world demography of type 2 diabetes**, A review Article,[1]University of Aarhus, Århus, Denmark,[2]Novo Nordisk Scandinavia, Malmö, Sweden[3]Novo Nordisk, Bagsværd, Denmark, Correspondence to Anders Green, Department of epidemiology and Social Medicine, University of Aarhus, Vennelyst Boulevard 6, DK-8000 Århus C, Denmark. Received: 15 May 2002; Revised: 1 August 2002; Accepted: 16 September 2002

15. World Health Organisation. Obesity: Preventing and Managing the Global Epidemic: Report of the WHO Consultation of Obesity. Geneva: World Health Organisation, 1997.

16. National Center for Health Statistics Health, United States, 2005 With Chartbook on Trends in the Health of Americans Hyattsville, Maryland: 2005

17. Cynthia L. Leibson, PHD[1], David F. Williamson, PHD[4], L. Joseph Melton, III, MD[1], Pasquale J. Palumbo, MD[3], Steven A. Smith, MD[2], Jeanine E. Ransom, BS[1], Peter L. Schilling, MS[1] and K. M. Venkat Narayan, MD[4] , **Temporal Trends in BMI Among Adults With Diabetes, Epidemiology/Health Services/Psychosocial Research Original Article**, Department of Health Sciences Research, Mayo Clinic, Rochester, Minnesota [2] Department of Internal Medicine, Mayo Clinic, Rochester, Minnesota [3] Department of Internal Medicine, Mayo Clinic, Scottsdale, Arizona [4] Division of Diabetes Translation, Centers for Disease Control and Prevention, Atlanta, Georgia

18. Loren Cordain[1], GK1. Boyd Eaton[2], Jennie Brand Miller[3], Staffan Lindeberg[4] and Clark Jensen[5], An evolutionary analysis of the aetiology and pathogenesis of juvenile-onset myopia 1 Department of Health and Exercise Science, Colorado State University, Fort Collins, Colorado, USA 2 Departments of Radiology and Anthropology, Emory University, Atlanta, Georgia, USA 3 Department of Biochemistry, University of Sydney, New South Wales, Australia 4 Department of Community Medicine, University of Lund, Sweden 5 Jensen Optometrists, Grinnell, Iowa, USA

19. Williams, Roger, J., Biochemical Individuality: The Key to Understanding What Shapes Your Health

20. Lindsey F Masson, Geraldine McNeill and Alison Avenell;. Genetic variation and the lipid response to dietary intervention: a systematic review. American Journal of Clinical Nutrition, Vol. 77, No. 5, 1098-1111, May 2003

21. Eidenier, H., et al, A Manual for Metabolic/Nutritional Evaluation of the   SMA/25, CBC w/Differential and Related Tests, 1995 Rev 1: 20-25

22. Kalat,J.,W., Biological Psychology, 4th Edition, 1992

23. Frisancho, A., O., Human Adaptation A Functional Interpretation, University of Michigan Press 1989

24. Nugent. S. D., How To Survive on a Toxic Planet 2nd edition Alethia Corporation, 2004

25. Nugent. S. D., The Missing Nutrients 1st and 2nd editions Alethia Corporation, 2005

26. Shils ME;. *Modern Nutrition in Health and Disease*. Baltimore, MD: Lippincott/Wililams & Wilkins; 1998.

27. D; Sanders K; Kolybaba M; Lopez D;. Case-control study of phytoestrogens and breast cancer. *Lancet*. 350: 990-994.

28. Tham DM;Gardner CD;Haskell WL;. Clinical review 97: Potential health benefits of dietary phytoestrogens: a review of the clinical, epidemiological, and mechanistic evidence. *J Clin Endocrinol Metab*. 83: 2223-2235.

29. Barnes GK1;. The chemopreventive properties of soy isoflavonoids in animal models of breast cancer. *Breast Cancer Res Treat*. 46: 169-179.

30. Stephens FO;. The rising incidence of breast cancer in women and prostate cancer in men. Dietary influences: a possible preventive role for nature's sex hormone modifiers - the phytoestrogens (review). *Oncol Rep.* 6: 865-870.

31. Melissa Lee Phillips, Hunger hormone tied to learning www.the-scientist.com February 20, 2006

32. J. Kling, "Elusive ligand ghrelin could have numerous roles," *The Scientist*, June 10, 2002. http://www.the-scientist.com/article/display/13099/

33. GK1. Blackman, "The hunger hormone unharnessed, *The Scientist*, October 6, 2003. http://www.the-scientist.com/2003/10/06/30/1/

34. GK1. Diano et al., "Ghrelin controls hippocampal spine synapse density and memory performance," *Nature Neuroscience*, February 19, 2006. http://www.nature.com/neuro

35. Sabrina Diano http://info.med.yale.edu/bbs/faculty/sab_di.html

36. Robert Steiner http://depts.washington.edu/pbiopage/people_fac_page.php?fac_ID=30

37. A. J. van der Lely et al., "Biological, physiological, pathophysiological, and pharmacological aspects of ghrelin," *Endocrine Reviews*, June 2004. PM_ID: 15180951

38. M. Kojima et al., "Ghrelin is a growth-hormone-releasing acylated peptide from stomach," *Nature*, December 9, 1999. PM_ID: 10604470

39. V. G 4. Carlini et al., "Ghrelin increases anxiety-like behavior and memory retention in rats," *Biochemical and Biophysical Research Communications*, December 20, 2002. PM_ID: 12470640

40. N. Burgess et al., "The human hippocampus and spatial and episodic memory," *Neuron*, August 15, 2002. PM_ID: 12194864

41. K. Heyman, "Neurophysiology: Dust clearing on the long-term potentiation debate," *The Scientist*, May 23, 2005. http://www.the-scientist.com/article/display/15475/

42. Michael Cowley http://www.ohsu.edu/ngp/faculty/cowley.shtml

43. M.A. Cowley et al., "The distribution and mechanism of action of ghrelin in the CNS demonstrates a novel hypothalamic circuit regulating energy homeostasis," *Neuron*, February 20, 2003. PM_ID: 12597862

44. Christian Broberger http://www.neuro.ki.se/broberger

45. David E. Cummings http://depts.washington.edu/metab/faculty/Cummings.htm

46. Neel JV. The "Thrifty genotype" in 1998. Nutr Rev 1999;57:GK2±9.

47. Jennie Brand-Miller ;Kaye Foster-Powell ;Stephen Colagiuri The New Glucose Revolution She has authored several since by the way.

48. Foster-Powell K; Holt, SH; Brand-Miller JC; International table of glycemic index and glycemic load values: 2002. Am J Clin Nutr. 2002 Jul; 76: 5-56

49. Montignac. Michel, Eat Yourself Slim. Baltimore: Erika House, Book Publishers, May 1999.